ASSESSING UNIVERSAL HEALTH COVERAGE FOR BREAST CANCER MANAGEMENT

IS THE SERVICE AND FINANCIAL COVERAGE ADEQUATE FOR PREVENTIVE AND CURATIVE CARE?

PROFESSOR DR SYED MOHAMED ALJUNID

AND

DR AIDALINA BINTI MAHMUD

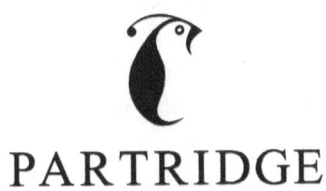

Copyright © 2021 by Syed Aljunid.

ISBN: Softcover 978-1-5437-6335-5
       eBook   978-1-5437-6336-2

All rights reserved. No part of this book may be used or reproduced by any means, graphic, electronic, or mechanical, including photocopying, recording, taping or by any information storage retrieval system without the written permission of the author except in the case of brief quotations embodied in critical articles and reviews.

Because of the dynamic nature of the Internet, any web addresses or links contained in this book may have changed since publication and may no longer be valid. The views expressed in this work are solely those of the author and do not necessarily reflect the views of the publisher, and the publisher hereby disclaims any responsibility for them.

Print information available on the last page.

To order additional copies of this book, contact
Toll Free +65 3165 7531 (Singapore)
Toll Free +60 3 3099 4412 (Malaysia)
orders.singapore@partridgepublishing.com

www.partridgepublishing.com/singapore

Contents

Acknowledgement xix

List of Abbreviations xxi

Chapter 1 Introduction 1

    1.1   Background 1
    1.2   Universal Health Coverage 1
    1.3   Research Problems 7
    1.4   Research Questions 8
    1.5   Research Objectives 9
    1.5.1   Main objective 9
    1.5.2   Specific Objectives 9
    1.6   Research Hypothesis 10
    1.7   Research Scope 10
    1.8   Research Importance 11

Chapter 2 Literature Review 12

    2.1   Introduction 12
    2.2   The Basics of Universal Health Coverage 12
    2.2.1   Brief history of UHC 13
    2.2.2   Dimensions of UHC 15
    2.2.3   The building blocks of the health system for UHC 16
    2.3   Monitoring Universal Health Coverage 18
    2.3.1   Measuring and Monitoring UHC: what and how 18
    2.3.2   UHC monitoring framework 20
    2.3.3   Service coverage indicators 24

2.3.4　Service coverage targets 27
2.3.5　Effective service coverage....................................27
2.3.6　Financial Protection Coverage.............................29
2.3.7　Building Blocks of the Health System................35
2.3.8　Composite Index...39
2.4　　Breast Cancer...40
2.4.1　Epidemiology of breast cancer.............................41
2.4.2　Pathology..42
2.4.3　Screening 43
2.4.4　Diagnosis 44
2.4.5　Treatment options...44
2.5　　UHC in Cancer 51
2.5.1　Service coverage...51
2.5.2　Financial protection coverage..............................52
2.6　　Conceptual Framework..53

Chapter 3　Research Methodology 55

3.1　　Introduction..55
3.2　　Component 1: Development of indicators
　　　 and targets...56
3.2.1　The compilation of service coverage
　　　 indicator criteria..57
3.2.2　The rationale of using quality performance
　　　 indicators (QPI) as service coverage indicators...61
3.2.3　Steps in developing the proposed
　　　 indicators for UHC in breast cancer
　　　 management..63
3.2.4　Proposed indicators for UHC in breast
　　　 cancer management...64
3.3　　Component 2: Measuring the extent of
　　　 UHC in breast cancer 73
3.3.1　Part 1: Determine the availability of
　　　 building blocks for UHC.....................................73
3.3.2　Part 2: Determine the effective service
　　　 coverage and the financial protection coverage....75
3.4　　Combined Data Analysis.....................................83
3.5　　Operational Definition of Terms 91

- 3.5.1 Service coverage for prevention 91
- 3.5.2 Service coverage for treatment 91
- 3.5.3 Catastrophic health expenditure 91
- 3.5.4 Impoverishment 91
- 3.5.5 Effective service coverage for breast cancer management 92
- 3.5.6 Financial protection coverage for breast cancer management 92
- 3.5.7 Age 92
- 3.5.8 Gender 92
- 3.5.9 Occupation 92
- 3.5.10 Education level 93
- 3.5.11 Marital status 93
- 3.5.12 Household 93
- 3.5.13 Single family 93
- 3.5.14 Nuclear family 93
- 3.5.15 Extended family 94
- 3.5.16 Composite family 94
- 3.5.17 Household income 94
- 3.5.18 Household food expenditure 94
- 3.5.19 Out-of-pocket expenditure (OOPE) 94
- 3.5.20 Combined OOP expenditure 95
- 3.5.21 Travel expenditure 95
- 3.5.22 Meal expenditure 95
- 3.5.23 Traditional and complementary medicine (TCM) 95
- 3.5.24 Breast cancer treatment 95
- 3.5.25 Capacity to pay 96
- 3.5.26 Poverty line 96
- 3.6 Research Ethics 96

Chapter 4 Results 97

- 4.1 Introduction 97
- 4.2 Proposed UHC Indicators for Breast Cancer Management in Malaysia 98
- 4.3 Availability of the Building Blocks of UHC 102
- 4.3.1 Leadership and governance 102

4.3.2	Health systems financing	104
4.3.3	Health information systems	105
4.3.4	Access to essential medicine	108
4.3.5	Health workforce	108
4.3.6	Service delivery	114
4.4	Effective Service Coverage	122
4.4.1	Mammogram screening	123
4.4.2	Surgery	123
4.4.3	Chemotherapy	124
4.4.4	Radiotherapy	124
4.4.5	Hormonal therapy	125
4.4.6	Targeted therapy	125
4.4.7	Palliative care	125
4.5	Financial Protection Coverage	129
4.5.1	Demography of respondents	129
4.5.2	Economic status of respondents	132
4.6	Catastrophic Health Expenditure	140
4.7	Impoverishment	145
4.8	Factors associated with catastrophic health expenditure and impoverishment	148
4.8.1	Association between sociodemographic and socioeconomic factors with CHE	148
4.8.2	Association between sociodemographic and socioeconomic factors with impoverishment	150
4.8.3	Predicting factors for CHE and impoverishment	152
4.9	Composite Index of Universal Health Coverage for Breast Cancer Management	156

Chapter 5 Discussion 161

5.1	Introduction	161
5.2	Framework, Indicators and Targets for the UHC Monitoring for Breast Cancer Management in Malaysia	161
5.3	Availability of the Building Blocks of the Health System for UHC	163

5.3.1 Leadership and governance 163
5.3.2 Health systems financing 164
5.3.3 Health information systems 167
5.3.4 Access to essential medicine 169
5.3.5 Health workforce 170
5.3.6 Health service delivery 171
5.4 Service Coverage for Breast Cancer Management 172
5.4.1 Mammogram screening 173
5.4.2 Initial treatment 173
5.4.3 Chemotherapy 174
5.4.4 Radiotherapy 174
5.4.5 Hormone therapy 175
5.4.6 Targeted therapy 175
5.4.7 Palliative care 176
5.5 Financial Protection Coverage for Breast Cancer Management 178
5.5.1 Sample size 178
5.5.2 Response rate 179
5.5.3 Sampling method 179
5.5.4 Respondent sociodemographic status 180
5.5.5 Respondent socioeconomic status 182
5.6 Catastrophic Health expenditure 188
5.7 Impoverishment 189
5.8 Factors Associated with CHE and Impoverishment Among Breast Cancer Patients 190
5.9 Predictive Factors of CHE and Impoverishment 195
5.10 UHC Index of Breast Cancer Management 196
5.11 Overall Results Interpretation 198
5.12 Limitations of this Study 200
5.12.1 Study design 200
5.12.2 Study location 201
5.12.3 Study population 202
5.12.4 Data collection methods 203
5.12.5 Study results 206
5.13 Strengths of This Study 206

Chapter 6 Conclusion and Recommendations 208

    6.1   Conclusion 208
    6.2   Recommendations for Future Research 209
    6.3   Policy implications based on this study 210

References 211

Appendix A 1   Indicators for UHC Monitoring (USAID July 2012) 243

Appendix A 2   Indicators for Service Coverage (USAID September 2012) 245

Appendix A 3   Indicators for Service Coverage (WHO & WBG 2014) 249

Appendix A 4   Indicators for UHC Monitoring (WHO & WBG 2015) 253

Appendix A 5   NICCQ Indicators 257

Appendix A 6   NICE Indicators 259

Appendix A 7   EUSOMA Indicators 261

Appendix A 8   Indicators for Health System Governance 263

Appendix A 9   Indicators for Health Systems Financing 265

Appendix A 10   Indicators for HISPIX 267

Appendix A 11   Indicators for Essential Medicines 269

Appendix A 12   Malaysian National Essential Medicine List (2014) Compared to The WHO Essential Medicines List (2013, 2015) 271

Appendix A 13	Sources, Indicators and Targets for Health Workforce	275
Appendix A 14	Indicators for Health Service Delivery	277
Appendix B 1	Patient Information Sheet (Bahasa Malaysia)	281
Appendix B 2	Patient Information Sheet (English)	283
Appendix C 1	Data Collection Form	285
Appendix C 2	Questionnaire	287

List of Tables

Table 2.1 Health expenditure targets 36

Table 3.1 UHC service coverage indicator criteria 60

Table 3.2 Effective coverage metrics 61

Table 3.3 Adherence of QPI to the criteria for UHC monitoring indicators 62

Table 3.4 Adherence to the criteria for effective service coverage 63

Table 3.5 Organizations with performance measurement systems 65

Table 3.6 Final Measures as Harmonized by ASCO/NCCN and CoC and Endorsed by the National Quality Forum 66

Table 3.7 Quality performance indicators for breast cancer, Malaysia 68

Table 3.8 Quality performance indicators for palliative care 69

Table 3.9 Quality performance indicators for palliative care 70

Table 3.10 Targets for UHC indicators 72

Table 3.11 Service readiness for breast cancer management 74

Table 3.12 Sample size options for service coverage.................77

Table 3.13 Sample size options for financial coverage...............79

Table 3.14 Summary of UHC index score..................................90

Table 4.1 Malaysian population based on year and gender.......97

Table 4.2 Proposed indicators for effective service coverage for breast cancer management.....................................98

Table 4.3 Availability of policy index..103

Table 4.4 Total General Government Health Expenditure (GGHE) as percentage of General Government Expenditure (GGE) 1997 -2015........................105

Table 4.5 HISPIX Malaysia..106

Table 4.6 Number of clinical specialists in Malaysia................109

Table 4.7 Percentage of increase in number of medical personnel 2008-2014...109

Table 4.8 Percentage of increase in number of specialist doctors per 10,000 population, 2009-2013..............................110

Table 4.9 Ratio of medical professionals in cancer management 2010-2015 per 10,000 population......................110

Table 4.10 Allied health professionals in cancer management 2010-2015...111

Table 4.11 Regional distribution of medical workforce per 10,000 population 2010-14..113

Table 4.12 Distribution of workforce according to sex (2011, 2013-14) 113

Table 4.13 Number of clinical specialists in MOH who gained postgraduate qualifications in five major disciplines (2009 -2013) 114

Table 4.14 Service-specific availability for breast cancer management at various levels of service 118

Table 4.15 Public and private facilities with breast cancer related services 119

Table 4.16 Specific service readiness for breast cancer management 122

Table 4.17 Summary of effective service coverage for breast cancer 128

Table 4.18 Demography of respondents 130

Table 4.19 Summary of origin and residence of respondents 131

Table 4.20 Distribution of employment status 133

Table 4.21 Distribution of the types and categories of financial aid 134

Table 4.22 Distribution of average monthly household income 134

Table 4.23 Distribution of average monthly household income according to quintiles 135

Table 4.24 Distribution of monthly household income according to income groups 136

Table 4.25 Estimated mean income between the income groups 136

Table 4.26 Estimated monthly food expenditure according to income groups 137

Table 4.27 Estimated percentage of monthly food expenditure from total household income according to income groups 137

Table 4.28 Estimated monthly capacity to pay according to income groups 138

Table 4.29 Estimated monthly treatment expenditure according to income groups 138

Table 4.30 Estimated monthly TCM expenditure according to income groups 139

Table 4.31 Estimated monthly travel and meal expenditure in income groups 139

Table 4.32 Median estimated travel and meals monthly expenditure 140

Table 4.33 Distribution of CHE within household income groups 141

Table 4.34 Socioeconomic description of the households which experienced CHE 142

Table 4.35 Poverty impact from OOP expenditure on breast cancer 146

Table 4.36 Frequency and percentage of SES status impoverished households 147

Table 4.37 Summary of the association between respondents' sociodemographic and socioeconomic factors with CHE 149

Table 4.38 Summary of the association between respondents' sociodemographic and socioeconomic factors with impoverishment 151

Table 4.39 Multiple Logistic Regression for CHE 152

Table 4.40 Multiple Logistic Regression Model of predicting factors of CHE 153

Table 4.41 Multiple Logistic Regression for Impoverishment 154

Table 4.42 Multiple Logistic Regression Model of predicting factors of impoverishment 155

Table 4.45 Summary of the calculation for UHC composite index 157

Table 5.1 Comparison of median of income 184

List of Figures

Figure 2.1 The UHC cube 15

Figure 2.2 Framework for measurement and monitoring of the service coverage component of Universal Health Coverage (Framework 1) 21

Figure 2.3 Framework for selecting indicators to monitor service coverage. (Framework 2) 22

Figure 2.4 Results chain framework for monitoring health sector progress and performance (Framework 3) 23

Figure 2.5 UHC monitoring framework by the WHO Regional Office for the Western Pacific (Framework 4) 24

Figure 2.6 Framework for UHC composite index 40

Figure 2.7 Algorithm for treatment of operable breast cancer 45

Figure 2.8 Algorithm of locally advanced breast cancer 46

Figure 2.9 Conceptual framework for UHC monitoring 54

Figure 3.1 Study framework 56

Figure 4.1 Monthly OOPE for breast cancer against monthly income 143

Figure 4.2 Concentration curve of cumulative out-of-pocket expenditure versus cumulative income.......................... 144

Figure 4.3 Monthly OOPE for breast cancer against monthly CTP 145

Figure 5.1 Financial protection, service coverage, and UHC index values 197

Acknowledgement

First and foremost, praises and gratitude be to Almighty Allah for all His blessings, for giving us the strength to complete this book.

We would like to express our sincere gratitude to academics and support staff of International Centre for Casemix and Clinical Coding (ITCC), UKM for their assistant and support in carrying out the research, which form the backbone of this book.

We would also like to express our highest appreciation to the Ministry of Health Malaysia for enabling us to conduct this study at the four tertiary public hospitals. We faced many challenges at the inception of the study and during the data collection phase. The health workers in these hospitals provide exceptional support and cooperation to make this research project a reality.

Dr Aidalina would like to acknowledge her husband, Anuarul Azhar Md. Yunus, and children Zarif and Zahin, for their patience and kindness during the conduct of the research. She would also like to thank Puan Rashidah Abdul Rashid, for her constant encouragement and prayers. A special thanks also to Dr. Norliza Chemi for the support given to her during the challenging times.

List of Abbreviations

CCI	Chronic conditions and injuries
CDR	Cytotoxic drug recombinant
CHE	Catastrophic health expenditure
CTP	Capacity to pay
DOSM	Department of Statistics Malaysia
EMRO	Eastern Mediterranean Regional Office (of the World Health Organization)
FANZCA	Fellowship of the Australian and New Zealand College of Anaesthetists
FRCR	Fellowship of the Royal College of Radiologists
FRCS	Fellowship of the Royal College of Surgeons
GDP	Gross domestic product
GGE	General government expenditure
GGHE	General government health expenditure
HCTM	Hospital Canselor Tuanku Muhriz
HISPIX	Health Information System Performance Index
HKL	Hospital Kuala Lumpur
HPJ	Hospital Putrajaya
HPP	Hospital Pulau Pinang
HQE	Hospital Queen Elizabeth
HRPZ II	Hospital Raja Perempuan Zainab II

HSI	Hospital Sultan Ismail
HSNZ	Hospital Sultanah Nur Zahirah
IQR	Inter-quartile range
M40	Middle 40 percent of the population
MDG	Millenium development Goal
MOH	Ministry of Health
MMED	Master of Medicine

INTRODUCTION

1.1 Background

This chapter starts with the background of universal health coverage (UHC) followed by the research problem, questions, objectives, hypothesis, justification and importance.

1.2 Universal Health Coverage

Universal health coverage (UHC) is defined as all people receive the health services they need, including public health services designed to promote better health (such as anti-tobacco information campaigns and taxes), prevent illness (such as vaccinations), and to provide treatment, rehabilitation and palliative care (such as end-of-life care) of sufficient quality to be effective, while at the same time ensuring that the use of these services does not expose the user to financial hardship (World Health Organization [WHO] 2015).

Universal health coverage is important for a country because through UHC there would be increased coverage of accessible health services and this could subsequently improve health status of the population. Improvement in health status was shown to give the largest gains among the poorer people (Moreno-Serra & Smith 2012). Universal health coverage is also important because it ensures people do not face financial difficulties in getting the health services or interventions they need. The financial difficulties in the context of UHC are catastrophic health expenditure and impoverishment. Catastrophic health expenditure is the point at which a household's out-of-pocket (OOP) expenditures are so high relative to its available resources that the household is required to forego the consumption of other necessary goods and services, while impoverishment is the condition when a person or household is pushed below the poverty line due to health expenditure incurred (WHO 2005; Xu et al. 2003). Universal health coverage has also been included into the post-2015 development agenda known as the United Nation's Sustainable Development Goals (SDGs) and every country should strive to achieve UHC by the year 2030.

To achieve optimum physical health, a person should be prevented from, and adequately treated against, communicable and non-communicable diseases (NCDs). One of the NCDs which warrants attention globally and locally is breast cancer. Breast cancer is the most common type of cancer among females in the Asia-Pacific, accounting for 18 percent of all cancer diagnoses (Youlden et al. 2014). Current trend shows that breast cancer incidence rate has been steadily increasing in all Asian countries, with an annual percentage increase of between 1.0% and 3.0% (Curado et al. 2007; Jemal et al. 2010; Parkin et al. 2005).

Based on the Malaysian National Cancer Registry Report 2007-11, female breast cancer in Malaysia accounted for 32.1 percent of all cancer among females in the country. Breast cancer patients in Malaysia present at a young age and at later stage of the illness compared to women in Western countries. A collaborative study between two tertiary academic hospitals in Malaysia and

Singapore found that between 1990 and 2007, approximately 50 percent of women were diagnosed before the age of 50 years, whereas in most Western countries such as the United Kingdom (UK) and Netherlands, 20 percent are diagnosed before age 50 years (Pathy et al. 2011). The National Cancer Registry of Malaysia between the years 2003 and 2006 reported that most of the patients with breast cancers presented Stage 2 (46.9%), and Stage 3 (22.2%), followed by Stage 4 (15.5%) and Stage 1 (15.5%). Similarly, between the years 2007 and 2011, the National Cancer Registry reported that that majority of the breast cancer patients presented at Stage 2 (37.0%), followed by Stage 3 (23.0%) and Stage 1 and 4 (20.0% respectively). As these results show, the incidence in stage 4 has increased in the most recent report period compared to the earlier one.

Over the years the Malaysian government has put in massive efforts in improving the detection and treatment of breast cancer. For example, the Healthy Lifestyles Campaign by the Ministry of Health which started in the early 1990s promoted awareness on breast cancer. In the year 2000s the Breast Health Awareness program was also launched to promote breast self-examination (BSE) to all women, to perform annual clinical breast examination (CBE) on women above 40 and mammogram on women above 50 years old. Additionally, from the year 2007 a subsidy program for mammogram screening by the Ministry of Women, Family and Community Development was made available, where women could either undergo screening mammogram for free or pay a minimal fee of RM50 based on their monthly income. As of 2016, the services by specialised breast surgeons were available in eight major government hospitals and two academic medical centres (the Universiti Malaya Medical Centre (UMMC) and Hospital Cancelor Tuanku Muhriz, previously known as the Universiti Kebangsaan Medical Centre (UKMMC)). Many more efforts in managing cancer were planned and detailed in the National Strategic Action Plan for Cancer Control Programs (NSPCCP) 2016-2020 (MOH 2015b).

Despite good progress in facility development for cancer treatment in Malaysia, accessibility to such services was still a major issue especially for those living in rural areas (Ministry of Health 2015b). Before a patient could get the appropriate treatment the patient would need to follow a certain chain of events, such as being seen by a doctor at the community clinic before being referred to the district hospital, then to the state hospital and lastly to a hospital which has oncology services (MOH 2015b). These multiple steps or chain of events often result in treatment delays.

Additionally, there is currently no known comprehensive studies on the the extent of financial difficulties faced by breast cancer patients in Malaysia. Information on financial difficulties of patients including breast cancer patients were commonly identified though newspaper articles. For example, between the years 2015 and 2016 there were five Bahasa Malaysia newspaper articles found online which featured individual breast cancer patients who had financial difficulties. These were of two elderly women aged 78 and 60 years old, and three younger women aged 33, 42 and 46 years old. The 78-year-old lady was bed-bound and taken care of by her 51-year-old mentally disabled son (Anon 2016a); while the 60-year-old patient was cared for by her elderly husband who did odd-jobs in his village in Kuala Pilah and had to travel to Hospital Kuala Lumpur monthly for treatment that cost them RM 150 per trip (Anon. 2016b). The 33-year-old woman was a mother of three children who had to stop working after being diagnosed with metastatic breast cancer (Mohamad Shofi Mat Isa 2016). Similarly, the 42-year-old unmarried woman also had to stop working following the diagnosis of breast cancer (Mohamed Sahidi Yusof 2016). Lastly was the 46-year-old housewife from Ipoh whose husband was a construction worker without fixed monthly income and they had two children who each suffered from asthma and heart disease. This family claimed that their monthly OOP expenditure for health was about RM 2000 (Anon 2015). Surely these were the extreme cases of financial difficulties or they would not have been featured in the newspapers. Nonetheless, these articles highlighted the extent of the OOP expenditure that can be incurred by the patients, the distance travelled, the unemployment and loss of income, as well as the diversity of the family composition of cancer patients.

The lack of research in financial protection coverage among cancer patients is also present in the neighboring countries. Regionally, there is only one study on catastrophic health expenditure (CHE) and impoverishment among cancer patients, which is the ASEAN Costs in Oncology (ACTION) study, carried out in the year 2012 and published in 2015. The results of the ACTION study involved eight ASEAN countries Cambodia, Indonesia, Laos, Malaysia, Myanmar, the Philippines, Thailand and Vietnam. Results showed that overall, about 48 percent of cancer patients of various cancer types experienced CHE one year after being diagnosed. For breast cancer the study showed that financial difficulty was experienced by approximately 60 percent of patients (ACTION Study Group 2015).

For a country to achieve UHC status by the year 2030, efforts are required to overcome the shortfalls in service coverage and financial protection coverage particularly for cancer. These efforts should be tailored to the country's technical and financial abilities in tandem with UHC concept of progressive realization of coverage according to a country's situation.

In terms of service coverage, a country must focus on the provision of effective service coverage. Effective service coverage means that people who need health services obtain them in a timely manner and at a level of quality necessary to obtain the desired effect and potential health gains. High level of financial protection coverage is also important, which means that patients who seek health intervention do not experience financial catastrophe or fall into impoverishment.

Regardless of the efforts, a country's health system must have good building blocks which are leadership and governance, health financing systems, health information systems, essential medicines, and health workforce and service delivery (WHO

2010b). Additionally, to achieve UHC status by the year 2030, progress towards it needs to be monitored to ensure all efforts are on track. UHC experts have proposed that the progress towards UHC is monitored by the level of effective coverage of interventions and financial risk protection (Evans et al. 2012).

Several low and middle-income countries are reported to have achieved UHC. These countries include Columbia, India, Korea, Mexico, South Africa and Turkey (Organization for Economic Co-operation and Development [OECD]). Malaysia too has been cited has having achieved UHC in several publications between the years 2011 and 2015 (Chua & Cheah 2012; Ng 2015; Savedoff & Smith 2011; Wan, et al. 2014) although the legitimacy of these claims is subject to further discussion and one's interpretation of UHC.

At present there are several local studies which seemed to focus on parts or components of the more recent definition of UHC (Lim et al. 2014; Clinical Research Center [CRC] Malaysia). Unfortunately, a comprehensive study on the extent of UHC in Malaysia is still absent. In fact, a comprehensive study on the extent of UHC which involves major non-communicable diseases such as cancer is also absent both globally. The absence of such studies could be due to the complexity of translating the proposed monitoring methods into practical actions because country situations are very diverse in terms of epidemiology, health systems and financing, and levels of socioeconomic development. Nonetheless, these obstacles should not be deterring the attempts in measuring the extent of UHC, especially sinceWHO has proposed that each country identify the most relevant and appropriate health conditions to be used as monitoring variable, provided the monitoring frameworks and indicators conform to the internationally acceptable ones (Boerma et al. 2014a).

1.3 Research Problems

Malaysia has been cited as having achieved the status of UHC. Having achieved UHC would mean that everyone is able to get the health care they need of good quality and in a timely manner without having to face any financial difficulty in the process. Despite this claim of the UHC status, there have been reports in the local mass media of patients having difficulties in accessing the needed health care. This discrepancy between the claims and the reports warrants further exploration of the issue of whether Malaysia has indeed achieved UHC and if so, to what extent. This exploration should include that of breast cancer management in Malaysia.

Based on the projection of studies in cancer, the incidence of breast cancer is in the increasing trend of approximately three percent per year in the Asian region. In Malaysia, national data show that breast cancer is already the most common cancer among women. Results of local studies also show that the incidence of breast cancer in Malaysia has been increasing among younger women and they are diagnosed at later stages of the disease. The change in the demography of breast cancer patients from older women to increasingly younger women may lead to serious implications to Malaysia. This country may lose the contribution from this productive group of the population because these young female patients then could only provide limited economic contribution and limited child-bearing potential. If these patients are experiencing financial difficulties while undergoing treatment of cancer, the effects on the wellbeing of their households especially their young children, could be devastating. In spite of this disturbing situation, at present the prevalence of catastrophic health expenditure and impoverishment among breast cancer patients and their households is not clear. Therefore, the status of financial protection coverage among breast cancer patients in Malaysia must be investigated.

Extensive efforts in the prevention and treatment of breast cancer in Malaysia since the 1990s by the government are commendable. Numerous awareness campaigns on breast cancer, screening programs and curative treatment have been made available over the years. However, to date, only one study has been carried out to determine the extent of quality in curative treatment of breast cancer in the country. No known study on the overall effective service coverage of breast cancer management is available; hence this necessitates the conduct of such a research.

The target for achieving the UHC status is the year 2030, as set by the United Nations in the Sustainable Development Goals. Many countries have indicated that efforts towards achieving this deadline are in progress. These efforts include strengthening the building blocks of the health systems of the countries. These endeavors need to be monitored so that any delays or shortcomings can be addressed appropriately and in a timely manner. However, based on available literature and reports, the major obstacle in monitoring these efforts is the absence of UHC framework, indicators and study tools for non-communicable diseases including cancer. Therefore, if the extent of UHC in breast cancer management is to be determined in Malaysia because of its high disease and economic burden to the country, then there is an urgent need to propose the associated UHC framework, indicators and study tools.

1.4 Research Questions

Based on the abovementioned research problems, this study presents the following research questions:

a. What is the suitable framework, indicators and targets to assess the extent UHC of breast cancer management?

b. What is the current level of availability of the building blocks of Malaysian health system in breast cancer management?
c. What is the current extent of effective service coverage for breast cancer management?
d. What is the current extent of financial protection coverage for breast cancer management?
e. What are the factors associated with, and predictors of, financial protection among breast cancer patients?
f. What is the extent of the UHC status (in terms of index score of UHC) in breast cancer management in this country?

1.5 Research Objectives

1.5.1 Main objective

The main objective of this study was to assess the extent of UHC status of breast cancer management in Malaysia.

1.5.2 Specific Objectives

The specific objectives of this study were to:

a. develop the framework, indicators and targets for assessing the extent of UHC of breast cancer management in Malaysia from the currently available criteria and indicators,
b. determine if the building blocks of the Malaysian health system are available, including that for breast cancer management
c. determine the extent of effective service coverage in breast cancer management,
d. determine the extent of financial protection coverage among breast cancer patients and their households,

e. determine the associating and predicting factors of catastrophic health expenditure and impoverishment among breast cancer patients and their households, and
f. calculate the composite index score of UHC in breast cancer management.

1.6 Research Hypothesis

In this research, it is hypothesised that

a. the building blocks of a strong health system are available, including that for breast cancer management,
b. the effective service coverage for breast cancer management is high,
c. the financial protection coverage is moderate,
d. the availability of financial aid is the significant factor associated with, and predictive of, catastrophic health expenditure and impoverishment among breast cancer patients, and the composite index score of UHC is moderate.

1.7 Research Scope

Universal health coverage is a concept which has been conventionally applied to a country's entire health system and service. Therefore, the frameworks, indicators and targets of UHC which are currently available are tailored for the scope of the whole health system of a country.

However, the scope of this study was narrower. This study was focused on breast cancer management in Malaysia. This focused approach resulted in the development of monitoring framework, indicators and targets which were specific for breast cancer. Subsequently, the framework, indicators and targets were applied on hospital-based data to determine the extent of UHC in breast cancer management in Malaysia. The results were then used in the UHC composite index framework and formula by Wagstaff et al. (2016) to deduce the composite index score for UHC of breast cancer.

1.8 Research Importance

Up until 2015, UHC monitoring on non-communicable diseases were limited globally, particularly for cancer due to the unavailability of the associated frameworks, indicators and targets of assessment. This study adapted these currently available frameworks, indicators and targets to propose a framework, indicators and targets for breast cancer management in Malaysia. It was anticipated that the current study would be a precedent of more studies in monitoring the progress of UHC among other non-communicable diseases.

The execution of this study was at an opportune time as Malaysia aspired to achieve 'developed' country status by 2020 and Malaysia's strive in achieving UHC and providing the best health care services to the people. The results from this study may contribute to the current knowledge in the development of frameworks, indicators and targets in the context of UHC monitoring; incite interest in developing and refining suitable indicators for monitoring of UHC achievements; and provide the baseline data for future studies and monitoring of UHC progress.

Ultimately this study may provide a preliminary overview of the extent of UHC in terms of effective service coverage and financial protection coverage in breast cancer management in Malaysia. To date, this study was the first of its kind in the country.

II LITERATURE REVIEW

2.1 Introduction

UHC's monitoring framework, indicator criteria and targets are discussed in this chapter. The building blocks of the health system needed to achieve UHC and breast cancer epidemiology are also reviewed. This chapter also delineates the gaps in knowledge on UHC in cancer and concludes with the conceptual framework for UHC in breast cancer management in Malaysia

2.2 The Basics of Universal Health Coverage

This first section discusses the brief history of UHC, the dimensions of UHC and the building blocks of a health system needed to achieve UHC.

2.2.1 Brief history of UHC

The idea of UHC began with the Primary Health Care (PHC) in 1960s. During that time, China, Tanzania, Sudan and Venezuela initiated successful programs to deliver basic health services covering poor rural populations (Bennett, 1979; Benyoussef & Christian, 1977). These programs came to be known as "primary health care" or PHC. Consequently, the World Health Organization (WHO) and the United Nations Children's Fund (UNICEF) used this concept of PHC to propose an equitable, accessible and affordable delivery of healthcare services in developing countries, emphasizing on prevention while still providing appropriate curative services. Finally, in 1978, the Declaration of Alma-Ata officially adopted primary health care (PHC) as the means for healthcare service for all countries. The approach involved multiple sectors (agriculture, education, women's groups, youth groups and ministers of religion). Goals and targets were then set for Achieving Health for All by the Year 2000 (WHO, 1981).

However, in the late 1980s and 1990s emphasis was placed on reducing government involvement in all aspects of society as market forces became the dominant model for service delivery. Governments of resource-poor countries had to adopt the market-driven economic reforms if they were to receive foreign aid and debt relief. Healthcare sector played the role of the sole provider in improving health, while other sectors were given little recognition, an approach which became known as Health Sector Reform (World Bank's World Development Report of 1993). Additionally, this Reform emphasized on using the private sector to deliver healthcare services while reducing or removing government services. As a result, user pays, cost recovery, private health insurance and public–private partnerships became the focus of most countries. Consequently, in the year 2000 when the Alma Ata Declaration was supposed to achieve its goals, many countries were in distraught because health care was not accessible to many of their population. Many people became impoverished due to the high out-of-pocket expenditure because of privatization of many health care providers.

Between the years 2000 to 2015, the United Nations developed the Millennium Development Goals (MDGs), which became the blueprint for the countries to address the issues of extreme poverty, healthcare and universal primary education. In September 2015, after the end of the MDG era, the United Nations declared a new set of blueprints known as the Sustainable Development Agenda. This agenda consisted of 17 goals known as the Sustainable Development Goals (SDGs) with 169 targets to be achieved by the year 2030. The SDGs were under the purview of the United Nations Development Program (UNDP). Goal 3 of the 17 goals was on Good Health and Well-Being. This Goal 3 aimed to ensure healthy lives and promotion of well-being for all at all ages. Specifically, achieving Universal Health Coverage (UHC) was stated as Goal 3.8.

The SDG Goal 3.8 was stated as: "Achieve universal health coverage, including financial risk protection, access to quality essential health-care services and access to safe, effective, quality and affordable essential medicines and vaccines for all". For Goal 3.8, there were two indicators, SDG Indicator 3.8.1 and SDG Indicator 3.8.2. SGD indicator 3.8.1 stated: "Coverage of essential health services (defined as the average coverage of essential services based on tracer interventions that include reproductive, maternal, and new-born and child health; infectious diseases; non-communicable diseases; and service capacity and access; among the general and the most disadvantaged population)". In essence, this indicator 3.8.1 captured the service coverage dimension of UHC (that everyone should receive the health services they need).

On the other hand, SDG indicator 3.8.2 stated: "Proportion of population with large household expenditures on health as a share of total household expenditure or income". In essence indicator 3.8.2 captured the financial protection dimension of UHC (use of health services should not lead to financial hardship).

2.2.2 Dimensions of UHC

There are three main dimensions of UHC: population coverage, service coverage and financial protection (WHO 2010a). These three dimensions represent the policy options a country can use to achieve UHC and are commonly depicted as the UHC cube (Figure 2.1). The current condition of a country's population coverage, service coverage and financial protection are depicted as the smaller blue cube. A country can choose to reform one dimension or more, but simultaneously reforming all dimensions could be challenging as additional resources may be required (Mathauer et al. 2009).

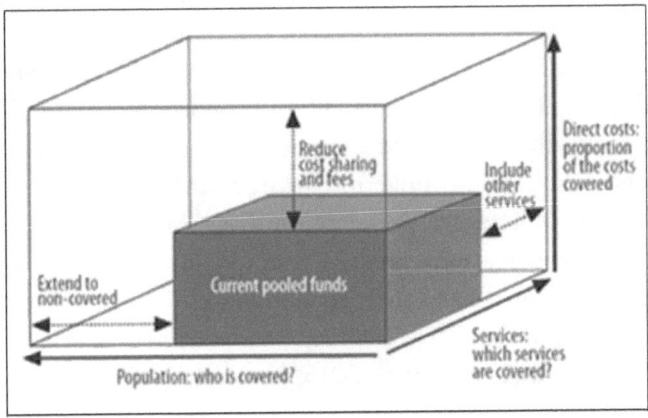

Figure 2.1 The UHC cube

The first dimension is the population coverage, which corresponds to the "breadth" of UHC cube. Population coverage is defined as the share of the population receiving a core set of health care goods and services under public programs and through health insurance. It includes those covered in their own name and their dependents (Organisation for Economic Co-operation and Development [OECD] 2017).

The second dimension is service coverage which corresponds to the "depth" of the UHC and basically refers to the range or collection of explicit services (sometimes referred to as benefits package) which are covered by pooled financing. Service coverage also includes the capacity of the system to provide the benefit package. The minimum health benefit package in a country depends on the availability of the country's resources, as well as the magnitude and distribution of health problems (Glassman & Chalkidou 2012).

The third dimension of the UHC cube is financial protection which corresponds to the "height" of the UHC cube. There are two aspects of financial protection: protection from catastrophic health expenditure (CHE) and protection from impoverishment due to health expenditure. In essence, financial protection prevents people from incurring high out-of-pocket (OOP) expenses on health care. Financial protection is usually in the form of pooled funds to spread the financial risks of illness across the population and allow for cross-subsidy from rich to poor and from healthy to ill and elimination of user fees. High proportion use of OOP for health expenditures can have a negative impact on the population: 1) it could discourage people from using health services, 2) it could cause them to disregard prescription drug therapies or postpone necessary investigations, and 3) it could force them to choose between their health and their economic well-being often referred to as catastrophic health expenditure and 4) it could cause a family to become poor (Guy Jr et al. 2015; Xu et al. 2007).

2.2.3 The building blocks of the health system for UHC

According to the WHO, for a country to achieve UHC, building blocks of the health system must be in place. These factors are leadership and governance, health systems financing, availability of essential medicines and technologies and enough capacity of well-trained, motivated health workers (WHO 2010b).

a. Leadership and governance

Available literature shows that adopting UHC is primarily a political rather than a technical issue (Greer & Mendez 2015; Stuckler, et al. 2010). So, to achieve UHC, firstly there must a solid commitment of the government in developing high-level policy goals and strategy for achieving these policy goals. Legal commitment is also a key factor in the realization of UHC, especially in establishing a comprehensive finance system because UHC implementation can be expensive especially at its early stages (Greer & Mendez 2015; Stuckler, et al. 2010).

b. System for financing health services

The second building block is the health systems financing, which includes revenue collection, fund pooling and purchasing. Having a sustainable and equitable form of revenue is crucial in UHC.

c. Availability of health information systems

The third building block is the health information system, which provides the foundation for decision-making and has four key functions: data generation, data compilation, data analysis and synthesis and data communication and use (WHO 2008). There must also be a mechanism in place so that information can be accessible to communities, health professionals and politicians.

d. Availability of essential medicines and technologies

The fourth building block is access to essential medicines. Essential medicines are always intended to be available within the context of functioning health systems, in adequate amounts, in the appropriate dosage, with assured quality, and at a price that individuals and the community can afford.

e. Enough capacity of well-trained, motivated health workers

There must be arrangements for achieving enough numbers of the right mix (numbers, diversity and competencies) of the workforce. Other factors which need to be addressed are payment systems and regulatory mechanisms to ensure distribution of workforce in accordance with needs. Additionally, there should be establishment of job-related norms, enabling work environments, and mechanisms to ensure cooperation of all stakeholders.

f. Service delivery

The last building block is service delivery. Service delivery is an immediate output of the inputs into the health system (health workforce, procurement and supplies, and financing). Concepts that have frequently been used to measure health service delivery are access, availability, utilization and coverage.

2.3 Monitoring Universal Health Coverage

In this section, monitoring of UHC in several countries up to the year 2015 is discussed. This is followed by a description of the basic concepts of measuring and monitoring UHC from the historical and technical perspectives.

2.3.1 Measuring and Monitoring UHC: what and how

Malaysia has been cited has having achieved the UHC status in several reports and publications. For example, a study by Wan et al. (2014) concluded that the modern public health care system in Malaysia with wide geographical coverage provided comprehensive care at minimal fees to the country's citizens qualifies Malaysia as country with UHC (Wan et al. 2014).

- Similarly, according to the authors of a report on the historical path toward universal health coverage of Sweden, Japan, Chile and Malaysia, Malaysia's historical path in reducing infant mortality rate, Malaysia can regarded as having achieved UHC (Savedoff & Smith 2011).

According to a document for the Global Network for Health Equity, Malaysia's achievement of universal health coverage was due to the country's effective health system and health financing, which has a progressive distribution, relatively small average household out-of-pocket payments were especially for poorer households and extensive networks of public health facilities (Ng 2015).

Finally, a local study used the WHO Health Financing Strategy for the Asia Pacific Region 2010-2015 as the framework to evaluate the Malaysian health care financing system in terms of the provision of universal coverage for the population. There were four indicators and targets used in this framework were: 1) total health expenditure at or less than 5% of the GDP, 2) out-of-pocket payment below 40% of total health expenditure, 3) comprehensive social safety nets for vulnerable populations, and 4) a national risk-pooled scheme for the population. Their findings showed that Malaysia has achieved all the targets in UHC health financing (Chua & Cheah 2012).

In other countries such as China, Thailand and Mexico prior to 2015, the measurement of UHC achievements were mostly on the efforts on expanding population coverage for health care (Wagstaff et al. 2013). This population coverage was either through social health insurance scheme or a national health service–type system that pools resources which then provides access to health services that are or close to zero-price at the point-of-use (Savedoff et al. 2012).

Another approach to measuring UHC was grounded on the rights-based approach. This approach started from the position that health is a human right (Backman et al. 2009). Based on this approach, countries which have endorsed the International Covenant on Economic, Social, and Cultural Rights (ICESCR) and the Convention on the Rights of the Child (CRC) were considered to have attained UHC. By endorsing these rights legally and morally, the leaders were bound to ensure the "highest attainable standard of health, encompassing medical care, access to safe drinking water, adequate sanitation, education, health-related information, and other underlying determinants of health." these approaches of measuring UHChowever, were deemed inappropriate by Wagstaff et al. (2016). Wagstaff argued that in a sense, everyone and most countries if not all, had already achieved UHC. Instead, Wagstaff proposed the measurement of the *depth* of the health coverage, referring to the amount umber of medical benefits received by an individual and what people pay in practice, and how affordable these payments are. There must also be equity in linking health care to the need and the quality of care, which includes making sure providers prescribe treatment that is appropriate and affordable.

In terms of how UHC is *monitored*, there were no standardized methods until after the year 2012. Between the years 2012 and 2015, several versions of the UHC framework and several indicators and targets were proposed which delineated how UHC was to be monitored (Boerma et al. 2014(a); Rockefeller Foundation Center, Bellagio 2012; WHO 2014; WHO 2016). These frameworks, indicators and targets are discussed in the following sections.

2.3.2 UHC monitoring framework

The following section will discuss the evolution of UHC framework and monitoring. As work and discussion on improving UHC monitoring at the global level is continually being carried out, the following description of UHC monitoring was current for the time frame during which this study was conducted (2015-2017). The discussion on this matter is crucial to understand the basics of the general UHC frameworks, indicators and targets.

These basic concepts will be adapted and adopted later in the proposal and development of the framework, indicators and targets for breast cancer management in Malaysia.

a. **Framework 1**

A UHC framework was first proposed in a report of a WHO meeting in Bellagio, Italy in September 2012 (Rockefeller Foundation Center Bellagio 2012). This framework for health service coverage addressed the priority health conditions. This framework referred to as Framework 1 in this study is shown in Figure 2.2. The foundation of this framework was the inputs and outputs of the health systems. The foundation cuts across all delivery areas. Inputs included financing, health work force, medicines and governance, while outputs included service availability and readiness, quality of care and utilization of services.

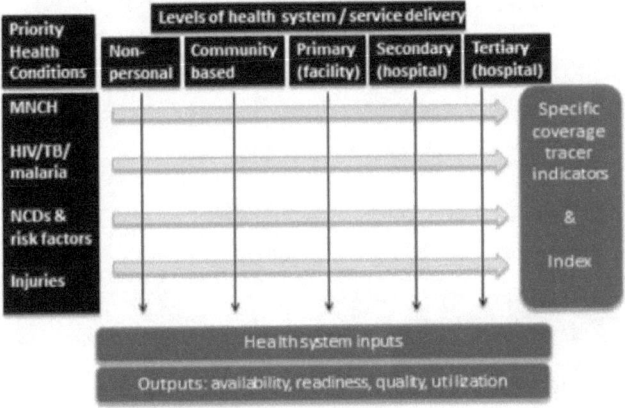

Figure 2.2 Framework for measurement and monitoring of the service coverage component of Universal Health Coverage (Framework 1)

b. **Framework 2**

In December 2013, the WHO and the WBG proposed detailed monitoring requirements at country and global levels

(WHO 2014). In that proposal, the framework for UHC monitoring (referred to as Framework 2 in this study) focused on only two discrete components of health system performance, and not three components as depicted in the UHC cube of the World Health Report 2010. These two components were: 1) the levels of essential health services coverage for the population and 2) financial protection coverage for the population with a focus on equity. Two measures of health interventions were proposed: 1) the set of interventions related to health MDGs and 2) the set of interventions related to chronic conditions and injuries (CCIs). This spectrum of services was then categorized further into two broad categories: 1) prevention and promotion; 2) treatment and care, as shown in Figure 2.3 below.

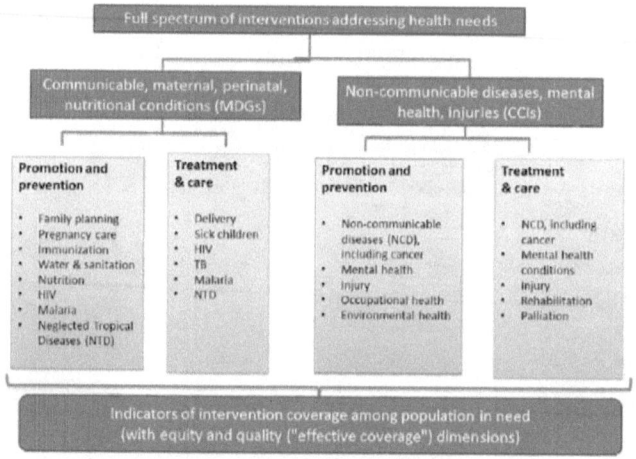

Figure 2.3 Framework for selecting indicators to monitor service coverage. (Framework 2)

c. Framework 3

In 2014, the WHO presented another framework for monitoring health system performance that can be used to track progress towards UHC (Boerma et al. 2014(a)). This framework is referred to as Framework 3 in this study and is shown in Figure 2.4.

This framework comprised of a results chain of inputs, outputs, outcome, and impact. Underlying the results-chain were the social determinants of health. Input and output factors helped explain the observed levels of coverage and are useful in identifying policy changes that might be needed to improve coverage. These input and output factors were also referred to as the building blocks of the health system. On the other hand, the outcome factor comprised of intervention coverage, financial protection coverage and health risk reduction. For intervention coverage, the authors proposed that its indicators should measure the health problems which were most relevant to the country. These indicators could be classified into different classes depending on: 1) the type of intervention (promotion, prevention, treatment, rehabilitation, palliative care), 2) the type of condition (related to MDGs, or related to NCDs/CCIs, 3) the characteristics of the target population and 4) the level of delivery of the interventions (from non-personal or population health to tertiary level care). Lastly, the impact in this chain comprised of mortality and morbidity rates by age, sex and cause. According to the authors, these impacts would be less suitable to monitor UHC because they were insufficiently specific to UHC and they were strongly affected by socioeconomic, environmental, behavioural, and other determinants of health (Boerma et al. 2014a).

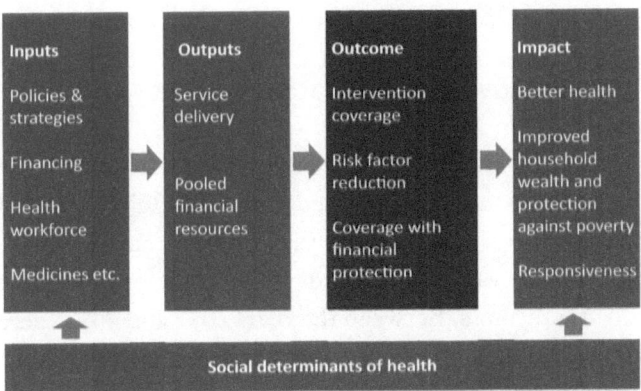

Figure 2.4 Results chain framework for monitoring health sector progress and performance (Framework 3)

d. Framework 4

In July 2015, the WHO Regional Office for the Western Pacific and the Asian Development Bank proposed yet another UHC framework, referred to as Framework 4 in this study (Figure 2.5). This framework tailored the measurement of progress on UHC specific to the Western Pacific Region (WHO 2016a).

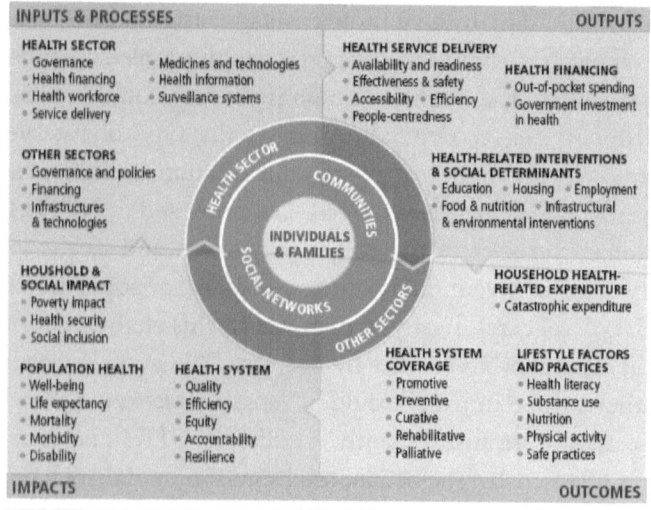

Figure 2.5 UHC monitoring framework by the WHO Regional Office for the Western Pacific (Framework 4)

2.3.3 Service coverage indicators

In this section, effective service coverage, its indicators and its targets are discussed. As discussed earlier, UHC progress should be measured using indicators. As the potential number and variety of indicators are vast, there needs to be a set of criteria for the selection of indicators. Between the years 2012 and 2015 there were several suggestions for the criteria of UHC monitoring indicators. There are four major documents about UHC monitoring which proposed sets of UHC monitoring indicators (Boerma et al. 2014a; Haas et al. 2012; WHO 2015).

The first two documents were reports by the USAID, published in July and September 2012. In these reports, two lists of potential service coverage indicators for UHC monitoring were presented. The first had 24 indicators while the second had 18 indicators (Appendices A1 and A2). The indicators were on maternal and child health, HIV treatment, TB treatment, vaccination coverage and malarial management. There was a category called quality, but there were no further details on it other than the phrase 'to be determined' (Haas et al. 2012).

The third document was entitled "Monitoring progress towards universal health coverage at country and global levels: Framework, measures and targets" by the WHO and the WBG published in the year 2014, where a list of intervention coverage indicators was proposed (Boerma et al. 2014a). In this list there were 19 indicators, which for the first time included the indicators on cancer (Appendix A3). Surprisingly however, there were no specific indicators on the prevention and/or treatment of other more common NCDs such as hypertension or diabetes. As for cancer, the prevention and promotion indicators were on cervical cancer screening, Human Papilloma Virus (HPV) vaccination and mammography; while for cancer treatment the indicator simply stated 'cancer treatment' without any details.

The fourth document was published in 2015; in the First Global Report on UHC. This report contained 13 indicators for UHC service coverage monitoring (WHO 2015). For each indicator, data on the primary data source, numerator, denominator and equity measurement were required. The indicators were also divided into two categories: 1) promotion and prevention category and 2) treatment, rehabilitation and palliative category. This was the first list of indicators which included hypertension, diabetes and cataract surgery coverage (Appendix A4).

Based on these four major documents on UHC monitoring indicators for service coverage, the evolution in the number and content of the indicators was noted. The number of indicators decreased from 24 to 13, and the indicators list also became more detailed in terms of description of the indicators over the years, with the one in 2015 even specified the numerators and denominators as well as how equity can be measured for each indicator. However, it was surprising to note that at this stage, emphasis on NCD monitoring was not as much as that for communicable diseases and maternal and child health.

The significance of NCDs as a challenge to the health and economies of all countries has been highlighted at the international level in the last several years. For example, the United Nations General Assembly on the prevention and control of NCDs in 2011 recognized the global burden and threat of NCDs to the economies of many member states in the 21st century. Additionally, in the Political Declaration following that meeting, the urgency and importance of NCD disease burden was acknowledged and efforts to overcome this burden were detailed (United Nations 2012).

Fortunately, the WHO 2013 Comprehensive Global Monitoring Framework subsequently included 25 indicators that countries can use to monitor their implementation of national strategies to prevent and control NCDs (WHO 2013a). Of these indicators, the most relevant indicator for cancer was the indicator to assess the proportion of women screened for cervical cancer. Other cancer indicators include the availability of the vaccine against HPV; availability of cancer medicines, technologies, and palliative care; proportion of premature deaths from cancer; and cancer incidence by type.

Surprisingly however, the indicators to monitor service coverage for cancer continued to be lacking in the following years. For example, in 2014 when Boerma et al. (2014a) from the WHO proposed indicators for service coverage in their framework for monitoring UHC, they included mostly the MDG coverage indicators and a small set of NCD-related indicators that are part of the global action plan for monitoring the NCDs. Nevertheless, none of these indicators was for cancer.

Similarly, in 2015 when the SDG replaced the MDG, indicators to monitor service coverage for cancer was limited. Among the 230 indicators of the 17 SDG goals, the only indicators which had some association to cancer was indicator number 23 which was "probability of dying between exact ages 30 and 70 years from any of cardiovascular disease, cancer, diabetes, chronic respiratory disease, [or suicide]", and indicator number 30 which was "current use of any tobacco product (age-standardized rate)".

At the end of 2015, the WHO published a document entitled "Tracking UHC: First Global Monitoring Report". In it, the WHO acknowledged that the set of core health indicators used offered no insight into health service coverage for NCDs. For this reason, the report then proposed a small set of potential UHC tracer indicators for NCD, which were hypertension treatment coverage and diabetes treatment coverage (WHO 2015). Yet, again, service coverage for cancer was not included.

2.3.4 Service coverage targets

The ultimate target of service coverage is 100% effective coverage, while for essential health services; the minimum target is 80% coverage. For conditions such as HIV infection, surgical conditions and mental health which the exact population is difficult to determine, statistical modelling may be able to assist in determining the denominator and the recommended target should be set at 80% or 90% (Boerma et al. 2014b).

2.3.5 Effective service coverage

As detailed earlier, the monitoring framework put forth by WHO and the WBG in 2013 highlighted two major components critical to assessing UHC progress namely service coverage and financial protection coverage for all people. For measuring service coverage, the concept of effective coverage was noted in the framework. In contrast to crude coverage, which focuses solely on intervention access or use, effective coverage is a measure that unites intervention need, use, and quality. The comprehensiveness of this metric makes it more suitable for monitoring UHC (Ng et al. 2014).

The WHO and the WBG defined effective service coverage as the proportion of people in need of services who receive services of good quality to obtain potential health gains (WHO 2015). Another definition of effective coverage was the fraction of potential health gain that is delivered to the population through the health system, given its capacity (Ng et al. 2014).

Boerma et al. (2014a) defined effective coverage as people who need health services obtain them in a timely manner and at a level of quality necessary to obtain the desired effect and potential health gains. Effective coverage is imputed as people with normal test results (i.e. received treatment and successfully treated) divided by people in need of the intervention (which includes people on treatment irrespective of test results, and people with positive test and not on treatment).

There are three components of effective service coverage: need, use, and quality (Ng et al. 2014). These three components need to be measured in a consistent and collective way. Need is whether an individual would benefit from receiving a specific health intervention. Use reflects whether an individual who needs the intervention, received or used a specific intervention. Quality captures whether a specific intervention conferred the health gain or protection it was supposed to or if the health benefit was received by the individual who obtained that intervention. The authors also believed that effective coverage was a very flexible metric that can easily be adapted for different contexts and assessed at different administrative levels. Therefore, it is an appropriate indicator for tracking progress and benchmarking performance.

2.3.6 Financial Protection Coverage

Financial protection is the protection against the economic impact of ill health, which are catastrophic health expenditure (CHE) and impoverishment (Kutzin 2008; WHO 2000). The key to financial protection is to prevent people from using their own money and pay out-of-pocket (OOP) for health expenditure. High OOP expenditure on health can lead to CHE. CHE is the official indicator for monitoring of UHC financial protection among the Sustainable Development Goals (Indicator 3.8.2).

The WHO defined OOP on health as direct payments made by individuals to health care providers at the time-of-service utilization. This excludes any prepayment for health services, for example in the form of taxes or specific insurance premiums or contributions and, where possible, net of any reimbursements to the individual who made the payments (WHO 2017).

The WBG defined OOP on health as any health expenditure of the household, including gratuities and in-kind payments, to health practitioners and suppliers of pharmaceuticals, therapeutic appliances and other goods and services whose primary intent is to contribute to the restoration or enhancement of the health status of individuals or population groups. It is a part of private health expenditure (The World Bank 2013).

The Organisation for Economic Co-operation and Development (OECD) defined household OOP as cost-sharing, self-medication and other expenditure paid directly by private households, irrespective of whether the contact with the health care system was established on referral or on the patient's own initiative (OECD 1991).

a. Financial protection indicators

For financial protection in health there are two commonly used general indicators: the incidence of catastrophic health expenditure (CHE) and the incidence of impoverishment due to out-of-pocket health payments.

There are two approaches in determining if a household faces CHE. The first approach considers the OOP payments as a proportion of income (X), which is OOP/X. Thresholds for OOP/X which could render a household into CHE varied from 2.5% to 15% (Wagstaff & van Doorslaer 2003). The use of income as the denominator could be problematic as households with savings or larger income will not be too affected by their OOP health expenditure even if the amount of the OOP exceeded the CHE threshold. The household with saving may finance their health care from their savings, whereas the household having no savings must cut back on their current consumption to pay for health care. The household with saving would not experience CHE while the household without savings would. However, this difference would not be reflected if the ratio of OOP health expenditure to income was used because the ratio would be the same for both households (O'Donnell et al. 2007).

The second approach in determining if a household faces CHE considers the OOP payments as a proportion of household expenditure. If total household expenditure is used as the denominator, the catastrophic payments are defined in relation to the health payments budget share, i.e. the proportion of the household budget allocated for health care expenditure. However, a potential problem is that this budget share may be so low for poor households in low-income countries, that there is no allocation left for health care expenditure because all budget (available income) is used to buy items essential to sustenance, such as food. As a result, households that cannot afford to meet catastrophic payments are ignored. A partial solution is to define catastrophic payments not with respect to budget share but with respect to expenditure net of spending on necessities. Expenditure net of spending on basic necessities has been referred to as "nondiscretionary expenditure" (Wagstaff & van Doorslaer 2003) or "capacity-to-pay" (Xu et al. 2003).

The third approach considers OOP health expenditure as proportion of the expenditure net of spending on basic necessities. The amount of available funds net of spending of basic necessities is referred to as capacity-to-pay (CTP) or sometimes ability-to-pay (ATP). Some studies compute ATP as income less actual food spending (Wagstaff & van Doorslaer, 2003). Another method proposed by the WHO expresses CTP as effective income remaining after basic subsistence expenditure (Xu et al. 2003). Subsistence expenditure is defined as the average food expenditure of households whose food expenditure share is in the 45th to 55th range. Xu et al. (2003) defined OOP health expenditure as being catastrophic if a household's financial contributions to the health system exceed 40% of income remaining after subsistence needs have been met.

The threshold for CHE refers to the approximate level of spending beyond which the household is forced to sacrifice other basic needs, sell assets, incur debt or become impoverished. The threshold at which health payments become catastrophic range between 10% and 40% (Limwattananon, Tangcharoensathien & Prakongsai, 2007; Wagstaff & van Doorslaer 2003; WHO 2015). There is no established gold standard for choosing any approach mentioned and there has been considerable debate on the definition of household resources and the threshold level for CHE (Limwattananon, Tangcharoensathien, Prakongsai, 2007; Kimani et al. 2016). In general, if total household income is used as the denominator, the most common threshold is 10%. If capacity-to-pay is used, the threshold is 40%.

For impoverishment due to health expenditure, there are three approaches. The first, is the absolute approach using the international poverty line. This approach determines the number of people with expenditures net of OOP falls below an international poverty line (Wagstaff & van Doorslaer 2003). The second approach is the WHO approach using subsistence food expenditure instead of the international poverty line. This approach considers the number of people with expenditure net of

OOP below levels corresponding to subsistence food expenditure but with expenses gross of OOP above subsistence levels of food (WHO 2015). Lastly is the absolute approach using different international poverty line which considers the number of people with expenditures net of OOP below the international poverty line applied to the country according to its WBG income group classification (Flores et al. 2008).

There are two indices to capture the impoverishment effects of OOP health expenditure: poverty head count; and poverty gap and ratio. Poverty head count captures the number of households which became poor due to OOP health expenditure (Van Doorslaer et al. 2006; Wagstaff & Doorslaer; 2003 Xu & WHO 2005). The poverty gap measures the percentage of deficit from the poverty line among the households which have become poor due to OOP health expenditure, while poverty gap ratio measures the percentage deficit from the poverty line of households that have become poor due to OOP health expenditure as a proportion of all the households in the population (Van Doorslaer et al. 2006; Wagstaff & Doorslaer, 2003).

b. Financial protection targets

For financial protection, the target was set by the WHO and the WBG at 100% protection from both catastrophic and impoverishing health payments for the population as well as for the strata of the population (Boerma et al. 2014b).

c. Factors associated with CHE and impoverishment

There are several factors associated with catastrophic health expenditure (CHE). Statistically significant association has been noted among older cancer patients and the experiencing of CHE (Choi et al. 2014; ACTION Study Group 2015). Results of studies also showed higher odds of experiencing CHE if households were having at least one member who was elderly (Somkotra & Lagrada 2009; Van Minh & Xuan Tran 2012; Van Minh et al. 2013).

Statistically significant higher odds of experiencing CHE were also found in households that have at least one member who was ill from any chronic non-communicable illness or hospitalized (Delavari, Keshtkaran & Setoudehzadeh 2014; Gotsadze, Zoidze & Rukhadze 2009; Shen & McFeeters 2006; Van Minh & Xuan Tran 2012; Ziller, Coburn & Yousefian 2006).

The gender of the household head was also associated with CHE. Results from studies showed that households headed by a male were found to be statistically significantly less likely to suffer CHE compared to households headed by females (Delavari, Keshtkaran & Setoudehzadeh 2014; Van Minh et al. 2013).

For a given value of health expenditure, the catastrophic impact of OOP depends on the food expenditure which in turn depends on household head's education. Households headed by someone with tertiary education were statistically significant less likely to suffer from CHE compared to those without education (ACTION Study Group 2015). Studies have also shown that there are statistically significant higher odds of experiencing CHE if the household head or members do not have paid work (ACTION Study Group 2015; Kumar et al. 2015). Lower income groups pay a higher share of their income compared to the higher income groups on health care therefore had significantly higher odds of financial catastrophe (ACTION Study Group 2015; Ruger & Kim 2007). Studies also showed statistically significant findings that households with family member enrolled in any insurance scheme had lower rates of CHE (Buigut, Ettarh & Amendah 2015; ACTION Study Group 2015; Van Minh et al. 2013).

The association between household location (rural versus urban) and the incidence of CHE also showed mixed results. Statistically significant higher odds of experiencing CHE were also noted if the household's residence was in the rural part of the country (Van Minh et al. 2013; Yardim, Cilingiroglu & Yardim 2010). Similarly, the odds of facing catastrophic health spending were higher for the city residents compared to non-city residents (Gotsadze, Zoidze & Rukhadze 2009).

Likewise, there are several factors associated with impoverishment. Households headed by females had statistically significant higher odds of becoming impoverished compared to those headed by males (Boing et al. 2014; Van Minh & Xuan Tran 2012). The odds of becoming impoverished also significantly lessened with the increase in the level of education (Boing et al. 2014; Kumar et al. 2015). Studies also showed statistically significant result that households in the poorest quintile were more prone to impoverishment compared to the richest quintile (Boing et al. 2014). The odds of being impoverished among people who did not have insurance were also higher than those who did (Boing et al. 2014; Van Minh & Xuan Tran 2012).

The association between having elderly members in a household location and the incidence of impoverishment also showed mixed results. Several studies show that having more elderly people was associated with statistically significant higher proportion of impoverishment (Kumar et al. 2015; Van Minh & Xuan Tran 2012). However, in Brazil, the odds of facing impoverishment were lower among households with elderly (Boing et al. 2014).

Households where there was at least one member with a chronic illness had a significantly higher odds of impoverishment compared to households without chronically ill member (Van Minh & Xuan Tran 2012). A study in China showed that households of four or more members in the rural areas were more likely to be impoverished than the urban ones (Kumar et al. 2015). On the contrary, a Vietnam study among rural population with chronic illness showed that having more people was significantly associated with lesser odds of impoverishment (Van Minh & Xuan Tran 2012).

2.3.7 Building Blocks of the Health System

In this section, six building blocks of the health system, their indicators and targets as proposed by the WHO are discussed. Countries can either choose to use these proposed indicators or modify the indicators according to the needs and situations in each country (WHO 2010b).

a. Indicators and targets for leadership and governance

There are two types of indicators for governance: 1) rule-based indicators and 2) outcome-based indicators (WHO 2010b). Rule-based indicators measure if the country has appropriate policies or strategies for health system governance. The indicators include the existence of documents such as the national essential medicines list or national policy for disease control. This class of indicators is called governance determinants.

On the other hand, outcome-based indicators measure whether the rules and policies are being effectively implemented, such as the availability of essential medicines at the health facilities. This class of indicators is called governance performance. As these outcome-based indicators are also part of the other building blocks of the health system, only the rule-based indicators for measuring health system governance are used in this study, as was undertaken by WHO in its guidebook (WHO 2010b).

There are ten proposed indicators to monitor leadership and governance in health. This set of indicators is called the Policy Index (WHO 2010b). For leadership and governance, each indicator is given a score of 0 if adequate governance policy does not exist or cannot be assessed; and 1 if an adequate governance policy is available. These indicators will result in a composite score of the governance policy index. The maximum score for the governance policy index is 10, but there is no set target or benchmark as to what value of the index score is good and what is not. The index score is to be monitored periodically and its trend over time would be used to assist the country identify key areas for improvement (WHO 2010b).

b. Indicators and targets for health systems financing

Core indicators for health systems financing are the: 1) general government expenditure on health (GGHE) as a proportion of general government expenditure (GGE), 2) total expenditure on health (TEH) as a percentage of gross domestic product (GDP) and 3) ratio of household OOP health expenditure to TEH.

Although GGHE as a proportion of GGE is a core indicator, is not widely used because countries claim that the target restricts the governments on their freedom to use their national budget (Mcintyre, Meheus & Rottingen 2017). Instead TEH as a percentage of GDP and ratio of household OOP health expenditure to TEH are more commonly used. It is a good indicator as it specifies the government health spending relative to the total economy, namely the GDP, as opposed to government health spending as merely a proportion of total government expenditure (Mcintyre, Meheus & Rottingen 2017). For health systems financing, there are targets are shown in Table 2.1 (Jowett et al. 2016).

Table 2.1 Health expenditure targets

Year	Source	Health expenditure targets		
		As share of GDP	As share of GGE	OOP/TEH
2009	WHO/WPRO SEARO	4-5% TEH		30-40%
	WHO/PAHO	6% TEH		
2014	McIntyre et al	5% GGHE		
	WHO/PAHO	5% GGHE		
2010	WHO	5-6% GGHE		15-20%
	WHO/EMRO		GGHE of 8%	

c. Indicators and targets for health information system

For health information system, the WHO proposed a Health Information System Performance Index (HISPIX). HISPIX is a summary measure of standardized indicators for assessing data quality and the overall performance of the health information system. It has six domains and 30 indicators. The six domains were: 1) health surveys, 2) birth and death registration, 3) census, 4) health facility reporting, 5) health system resource tracking, and 6) capacity for analysis, synthesis and validation of health data.

Most of these indicators are general in nature. Each indicator carries a score of 1 if the item is present and a score of 0 if it is not. This scoring system has a maximum score of 30, but there is no set target. Again, the index score would be used to assist the country in identifying key areas for improvement (WHO 2010b).

d. Indicators and targets for access to essential medicines

Access to medicines is included in the Millennium Development Goals under MDG 8, and specifically Target 8.E which states "in cooperation with pharmaceutical companies, provide access to affordable essential drugs in developing countries". Access has been defined as "having medicines continuously available and affordable at public or private health facilities or medicine outlets that are within one hour's walk of the population" (United Nations Development Group 2003). Therefore, the recommended core indicators for access to essential medicines are the average availability of 14 selected essential medicines and the median consumer price ratio of 14 selected essential medicines; in public and private health facilities.

In addition, the following indicators are recommended should a country wish to undertake a full pharmaceutical profile: 1) access to essential medicines/technologies as part of the fulfillment of the right to health, recognized in the constitution or national legislation; 2) existence and year of last update of a published national medicines policy; 3) existence and year of last update of a published national list of essential medicines; 4) legal provisions to allow/encourage generic substitution in the private sector; 5) public and private per capita expenditure on medicines; 6) percentage of population covered by health insurance and 7) percentage mark-up between manufacturers' and consumer prices (WHO 2010b).

e. Indicators and targets for health workforce

The health workforce can be defined as "all people engaged in actions whose primary intent is to enhance health" (WHO 2006). There are several indicators and targets for health workforce. During the MDG era, the World Health Report (2006) identified a minimum health worker density of 2.3 skilled health workers (physicians and nurses/ midwives) per 1000 population to attain high coverage (80%) of skilled birth attendance. However, in the SDG era, skilled health worker density of 4.45 per 1000 population corresponds to the attainment of 80% coverage (WHO 2016b).

The WHO recommends the following core indicators for health workforce: health worker density which is the number of health workers per 10 000 population; distribution of health workers – by occupation/ specialization, region, place of work and sex, to detect equitable supply, deployment and composition of human resources for health and the annual number of graduates of health professions educational institutions per 100 000 population – by level and field of education, to determine the supply and sustainability of workforce in the health services.

f. Indicators and targets for health service delivery

In general, the indicators for health service delivery can be grouped into four: 1) general service availability, 2) general service readiness, 3) service specific availability and 4) service specific readiness.

General service availability refers to the physical presence of delivery of services that meet a minimum standard. General service readiness refers to the general capacity such as infrastructure/ amenities, to provide health services. Service-specific availability refers to whether a specific service is offered. Availability is captured by the proportion of services offering a specific service and the density of the facilities offering the service per 10 000 population. Service-specific readiness refers to the capacity of health facilities to provide a specific service, measured through the presence of tracer items that include trained staff, guidelines, equipment/ supplies, diagnostic capacity, medicines and commodities. The tool by the WHO used to determine service availability and readiness called SARA (Service Availability and Readiness Assessment).

2.3.8 Composite Index

In 2008, the WHO and UHC experts proposed to combine the measurements of service coverage's prevention and treatment domains using the service gaps approach and subsequently to address the issue of equity (Boerma et al. 2008). In their proposal, service coverage was divided into prevention and treatment coverage. For each prevention and treatment domain, equal weights were given among the domains and within the domains. Therefore, to calculate composite service coverage index, the formula was as follows:

$$SC = \frac{\frac{[P1 + P2]}{2} + \frac{[T1 + T2 + T3]}{3}}{5}$$

where: SC = service coverage, P = prevention coverage, T = treatment coverage

The results were presented as a measure of the gap between maximum and actual coverage. For equity analysis, household income quintiles were used. Quintile 1 (Q1) represented the poorest 20% of households, and quintile 5 (Q5) represented the richest 20% of households. The difference between Q1 and Q5 was calculated to estimate the equity gap between the poorest and the richest. The ratio between Q1 and Q5 was then calculated to estimate the inequity ratio.

Subsequently in 2015, the WBG proposed another composite index which combined the service coverage measurement and the financial protection measurement. In this proposed composite index, a small set of tracer indicators for health services organized by prevention and treatment domains were combined into a composite measure, which was then combined with indicators of financial protection to provide a summary index of UHC as shown in Figure 2.6 (Wagstaff et al. 2016). In this framework, the service coverage and financial protection coverage were combined through a series of calculations which will be elaborated in the Methodology chapter of this thesis.

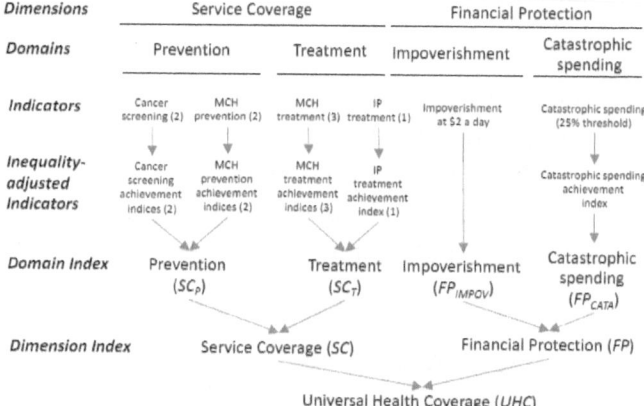

Figure 2.6 Framework for UHC composite index

2.4 Breast Cancer

The following sections will discuss 1) the epidemiology of breast cancer, 2) pathology of breast cancer, 3) screening of breast cancer, 4) diagnosis of breast cancer, and 5) treatment options of breast cancer.

2.4.1 Epidemiology of breast cancer

Based on the Global Cancer Incidence, Mortality and Prevalence (GLOBOCAN) 2012 results, breast cancer is the second most common cancer in the world and by far, the most frequent cancer among women with an estimated 1.67 million new cancer cases diagnosed in 2012 (25% of all cancers) (International Agency for Research on Cancer 2012). It is the most common cancer in women both in more and less developed regions with slightly more cases in less developed (883 000 cases) than in more developed (794 000) regions. Incidence rates vary nearly four-fold across the world regions, with rates ranging from 27 per 100 000 in Middle Africa and Eastern Asia to 96 in Western Europe. Breast cancer ranks as the fifth cause of death from cancer overall (522 000 deaths) and while it is the most frequent cause of cancer death in women in less developed regions (324 000 deaths, 14.3% of total), it is now the second cause of cancer death in more developed regions (198 000 deaths, 15.4%) after lung cancer. The range in mortality rates between world regions is less than that for incidence because of the more favorable survival of breast cancer in (high-incidence) developed regions, with rates ranging from 6 per 100,000 in Eastern Asia to 20 per 100 000 in Western Africa (International Agency for Research on Cancer 2012).

Within the Asia-Pacific region, about a quarter (24%) of all breast cancers are diagnosed approximately at a rate of 30 per 100 000. The greatest number were in China (46%), Japan (14%), and Indonesia (12%) (Youlden et al.2014). Incident of cancer cases were estimated to increase in Asia from 6 million in 2008 to 10 million in 2030 and cancer deaths from 4 million in 2008 to 7 million in 2030, considering the demographic changes in the population (Ferlay et al. 2010). The promotion of screening mammography and self-examination has led to the detection of the disease at earlier stages. Most OECD countries have adopted breast cancer screening programs as the most effective way for detecting the disease, although periodicity and population target groups vary (OECD/WHO 2016).

Age-standardized incidence and death rates of breast cancer per 100 000 populations ranged from 19.0 and 9.3 respectively in Lao PDR; to 65.7 and 19.6 in Singapore (International Agency for Research on Cancer 2012). There are more women under 50 years of age diagnosed with breast cancer at the time of diagnosis in the Asian region compared to the rest of the world, with the peak being in the 45-50-year age range within many Asian countries (Youlden et. al 2014), compared to a median of 55-60 years in most Western countries (Leong et al. 2010; Toi et al. 2010; Pathy et al. 2011).

Breast cancer patients in South East Asia are also diagnosed at more advanced stage of disease: 70 percent of cancers are diagnosed in locally advanced clinical stages, with overall 5-year survival being generally less than 50 percent (Sankaranarayanan et al. 2011). Advanced stage cancer is expensive to treat, treatment is almost always inaccessible, and many of those who can access treatment utilize their life savings and most likely not survive the disease.

According to the National Cancer Registry Report 2007-2011, breast cancer is the most common cancer in Malaysia, accounted for 32.1 percent of all female cases. The age-standardized rate (ASR) was highest in the 50-59 age-groups. The incidence of breast cancer was highest among the Chinese ethnicity with age-standardized rate (ASR) of 41.5 per 100 000 population, Indian (ASR of 37.1 per 100 000 population) and Malay (ASR 27.2 per 100 000 population). The percentage of breast cancer detected at stage I was 20%, stage II 37%, Stage III 23% and stage IV 20% (Azizah et al. 2016).

2.4.2 Pathology

Breast cancers can be divided into two main groups: the carcinomas and the sarcomas. Carcinomas arise from the epithelial component of the breast, which are cells that line the lobules and milk terminal ducts. Sarcomas are rare cancers that arise from the stromal (connective tissue) components of the breast. Carcinomas comprise most of all breast cancers, while sarcomas are rare. Breast cancer is staged according to the size of the tumour, number of lymph nodes involved and the absence or presence of metastasis. The American Joint Committee on Cancer (AJCC) Cancer Staging Manual using the Tumour, Node, and Metastasis (TNM) staging system is commonly used (Edge & Compton 2010).

2.4.3 Screening

There are three methods of early detection for breast cancer: breast self-examination (BSE), clinical breast examination (CBE) and mammography. While BSE and CBE can lead to downstaging of symptomatic disease, screening for asymptomatic disease by mammography will allow for detection of breast cancer in the earliest stage where cure is possible (Yip et al. 2008).

Mammography is non-invasive, relatively inexpensive and has reasonable sensitivity (72–88%) that increases with the age of the patient. Its primary advantage is the ability to detect tumours before they are clinically palpable. A large study by Weedon-Fekjær, Romundstad and Vatten (2014) amongst 638 238 Norwegian women aged 50 years to 79 years showed that modern mammography screening may reduce deaths from breast cancer by about 28 percent. In areas with screening (mammography) attendance of at least 70 percent, a reduction in breast cancer mortality by about 25 percent may be expected in women screened between ages of 50 and 69 years (Lauby-Secretan et al. 2015). Therefore, the WHO recommends that a well implemented screening program should achieve participation of at least 70 percent of the target group (International Agency for Research on Cancer 2002).

In Malaysia, currently there are opportunistic and targeted mammographic screenings, together with diagnostic mammograms at the request of doctors. The Malaysian Clinical Practice Guideline (CPG) on the Management of Breast Cancer recommends that for the general population, mammography may be performed biennially in women from 50 – 74 years of age, and breast cancer screening using mammography in low and intermediate risk women aged 40 – 49 years old should not be offered routinely (Ministry of Health 2010). However, Women aged 40 - 49 years should not be denied mammography screening if they desire to do so. The CPG also finds that benefit of breast self-examination (BSE) appears to be ineffective in reducing breast cancer mortality and thus recommends that BSE is for raising awareness among women at risk rather than as a screening method. For high-risk women, the CPG recommends screening to be done from the age of 30 years with both MRI and mammography as it is more effective than mammography alone.

2.4.4 Diagnosis

Triple assessment consisting of clinical assessment, imaging (ultrasound and/or mammography) and pathology (cytology and/or histology) for breast lumps is now an established method for the diagnosis of breast cancer in many parts of the world. If any one of the three methods yielded positive results, then breast cancer is diagnosed. However, all three methods need to be negative to exclude the diagnosis of breast cancer (Thomas et al. 1978; Khoda et al. 2015).

2.4.5 Treatment options

The Breast Health Global Initiative (BHGI) is an entity which provides evidence-based, resource-sensitive guidelines for breast cancer management in low- and middle-income countries (Anderson et al. 2008). Under the BHGI framework, a four-tiered system of resource allotment is used to establish prioritization schemes based on the level of existing resources (basic, limited, enhanced and maximal) and the stage of disease at diagnosis. Where available, basic surgery, low-cost generic drugs and radiation therapy are the basis of breast cancer treatment (Eniu et al. 2008). Mastectomy is the mainstay of treatment at the basic level. Endocrine therapy with generic drugs such as tamoxifen provides effective post-surgical treatment for tumours that are positive for oestrogen receptors (ERs). For oestrogen-receptor-negative cancers, systemic cytotoxic chemotherapy is effective but needs to be administered in a safe, sterile environment and requires monitoring for drug toxicity in the form of periodic blood chemistry profiles and complete blood counts. Radiation therapy allows for breast-sparing surgery and is used for chest wall irradiation after mastectomy and for the palliation of painful or symptomatic metastases.

Based on the Malaysian CPG of Breast Cancer Management, once the patient is diagnosed with early and invasive breast cancer (stages I-III) which is operable; and the patient consents to further intervention, treatment is initiated. Treatment algorithm for operable breast cancer and locally advanced breast cancer according to the Malaysian CPG is as shown in Figure 2.7, while for locally advanced breast cancer; the steps of treatment would vary depending on the operability of the breast cancer, as shown in in Figure 2.8.

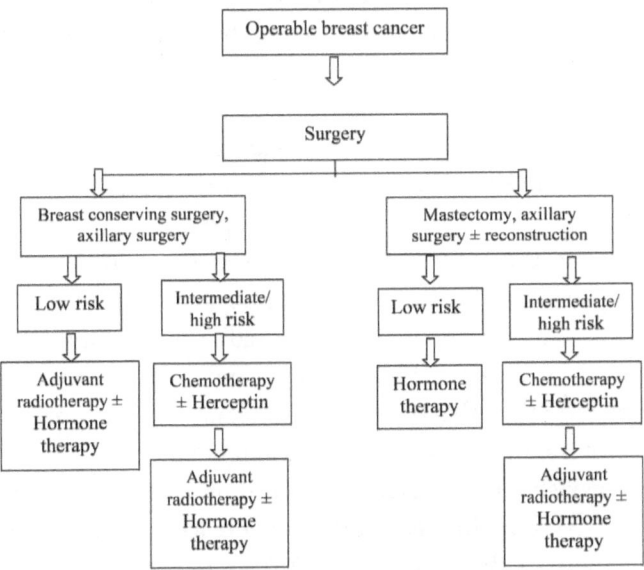

Figure 2.7 Algorithm for treatment of operable breast cancer

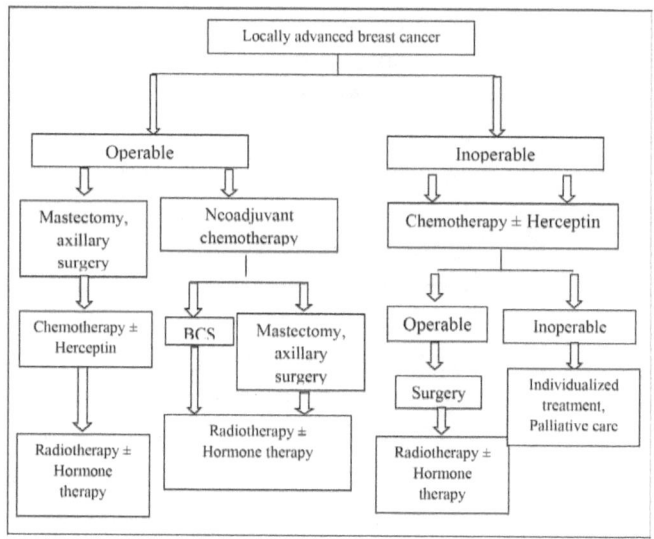

Figure 2.8 Algorithm of locally advanced breast cancer

a. Surgery

Surgery is considered the primary treatment for breast cancer. Goals include complete resection of the primary tumour with negative margins to reduce the risk of local recurrences, also for pathologic staging of the tumour and axillary lymph nodes to provide necessary prognostic information.

Surgery can either be mastectomy or breast conserving surgery (BCS). A total mastectomy involves complete removal of all breast tissue and is the most common surgical procedure in limited-resource settings. Breast conserving surgery (BCS) consists of wide local excision and followed by radiation therapy (RT) and assessment of axillary lymph node; and may be an option if adjuvant radiation therapy is available and women present with sufficiently small primary cancers (Eniu et al. 2008).

Surgery should be carried out until up to about 60 days post diagnosis (McLaughlin et al. 2012). In the Malaysian CPG on the Management of Breast Cancer (2010), it is not mentioned about the timing of surgery, but it states that newly diagnosed breast cancer patients should receive initial treatment within two months of presentation (Ministry of Health 2010).

The target for adherence to this 60-day duration (with its indicator being percentage of patients receiving their first definitive treatment for cancer within two months of a GP referral for suspected cancer) was 85% in England and 95% in Scotland, Wales and Northern Ireland (Cancer Research UK). The American Society of Clinical Oncology (ASCO) however, did not mention any target.

b. Systemic treatment

In general, systemic treatment in breast cancer includes cytotoxic chemotherapy, hormonal therapy, molecular-targeted therapy or a combination of these. Systemic treatment can be stratified into neoadjuvant (or pre-operative), adjuvant and metastatic settings, with each having a distinct goal. There are three main types of systemic treatment in breast cancer: chemotherapy hormonal therapy and molecular targeted therapy.

c. Cytotoxic Chemotherapy

Adjuvant chemotherapy eradicates micro-metastases, hence improves survival. Chemotherapy benefit is more pronounced in estrogen receptor (ER)-negative tumours (Berry et al. 2006; Early Breast Cancer Trialists' Collaborative Group, 2008). The Malaysian CPG on Breast Cancer Management (2010) recommends that adjuvant chemotherapy should be considered in all patients with early breast cancer.

Published clinical trials show a wide variation in the allowed time between surgery and adjuvant chemotherapy, ranging from 2 to 12 weeks (Bonadonna et al.1995; Cold et al. 2005; Farolfi et al. 2015; Ghany 2013; Levine & Steering Committee on Clinical Practice Guidelines for the Care and Treatment of Breast Cancer 2001; Lohrisch et al. 2006). Regardless of the initiation time, a systematic review and meta-analysis showed that overall survival decreases by 15 percent for every 4-week delay in initiation of adjuvant chemotherapy (Yu et al. 2013).

Neoadjuvant chemotherapy may be prescribed in locally advanced and large 'operable' cancers, to allow for achieving operability or decreasing the extent of surgery. The Malaysian Clinical Practice Guideline on Breast Cancer Management (2010) recommends that neo-adjuvant chemotherapy can be offered to patients with operable locally advanced breast cancer who are not suitable candidates for BCS at presentation to downsize the tumour to enable subsequent surgery.

d. Hormonal therapy

Following mastectomy, hormonal therapy decreases the risk of both invasive and non-invasive recurrences and reduces the incidence of second primary breast cancer (Senkus et al. 2013). There are two types of drugs which are commonly used - Tamoxifen and Letrozole.

Hormonal therapy is indicated in all patients with invasive early breast cancer and detectable oestrogen receptor (ER) expression (Berry et al. 2006; CPG on Breast Cancer Management, Malaysia 2010). In premenopausal women, Tamoxifen 20 mg/day for 5–10 years is a standard. For postmenopausal women with ER-positive early invasive breast cancer, should be offered an aromatase inhibitor, as their initial adjuvant therapy (National Collaborating Centre for Cancer UK 2009). Timing of hormonal therapy whether it should be taken together with radiotherapy or after radiotherapy, a study suggested that sequential tamoxifen treatment following radiotherapy is more effective than concurrent treatment (Jang et al. 2016).

e. Targeted therapy

Trastuzumab is a monoclonal antibody directed against the human epidermal growth factor receptor-2 protein (HER2). Trastuzumab is indicated as an adjuvant treatment for HER2-overexpressing breast cancer and for the treatment of metastatic HER2-overexpressing breast cancer. Trastuzumab use results increase in disease-free survival and reduction in risk of death (Gianni et al. 2012; Piccart-Gebhart et al. 2005; Romond et al. 2005; Slamon et al. 2011). The Malaysian CPG on Breast Cancer Management (2010) recommends that Trastuzumab be considered in women with HER-2 over-expressed or HER-2 gene amplified breast cancer having adjuvant chemotherapy.

f. Radiotherapy

After breast-conserving surgery, radiotherapy reduces recurrence and breast cancer death (Early Breast Cancer Trialists' Collaborative Group (EBCTCG), 2011). For patients who do not need systemic treatment, the interval between surgery and the start of radiotherapy should not exceed 8 weeks. For node-positive and high-risk patients receiving breast-conserving treatment, adjuvant chemotherapy should be administered prior to radiotherapy, but the delay of radiation should not exceed 20-24 weeks (Redda et al, 2002)

For post-BCS cases, radiation therapy is to be administered within 1 year (365 days) of diagnosis for women younger than age 70 years receiving breast conserving surgery for breast cancer, and the target is 90% adherence to this indicator (ASCO). The Malaysian CPG recommends that all patients with post-BCS should be offered adjuvant radiotherapy for both invasive breast cancer and ductal carcinoma in situ.

For post-mastectomy cases, the Malaysian CPG recommends that adjuvant radiotherapy should be offered to patients with more than four lymph nodes (N2 in TNM) and positive margin. However, newer evidence found that radiotherapy is also beneficial for 1-3 LN (N1 in TNM) involvement and T1-T2 tumours (Li et al, 2013; Recht et al, 2016).

g. Metastatic breast cancer

Advanced breast cancer (ABC) is a treatable but still generally incurable disease. The goals of care are to optimize length and quality of life. ABC patients can still be offered surgery, chemotherapy, hormonal therapy and targeted therapy. Studies have shown that surgical removal of the primary tumour was associated with a significantly longer survival time in patients with distant metastatic disease at diagnosis. (Ruiterkamp et al. 2009; Hazard et al. 2008). Taxane based chemotherapy is recommended in metastatic disease (Malaysian Clinical Practice Guideline on Breast Cancer Management 2010). Patients with ER-positive advanced breast cancer, who have been treated with chemotherapy, should be offered hormonal therapy. Targeted therapy should be offered early to all patients with HER-2+ ABC, except in the presence of contraindications to the use of such therapy.

h. Palliative care

The WHO defines palliative care as an approach that improves the quality of life of patients and their families facing the problem associated with life-threatening illness, through the prevention and relief of suffering by means of early identification and impeccable assessment and treatment of pain and other problems, physical, psychosocial and spiritual (WHO 2014). The WHO also detailed out the components of palliative care, some which are: provides relief from pain and other distressing symptoms, intends neither to hasten or postpone death, integrates the psychological and spiritual aspects of patient care, offers a support system to help the family cope during the patients illness and in their own bereavement and is applicable early in the course of illness, in conjunction with other therapies that are intended to prolong life, such as chemotherapy or radiation therapy, and includes those investigations needed to better understand and manage distressing clinical complications.

Similarly, the American Society of Clinical Oncology (ASCO) Clinical Practice Guideline uses the National Consensus Project definition of palliative care: palliative care means patient and family-centered care that optimizes quality of life by anticipating, preventing, and treating suffering.

The American College of Surgeons (ACoS) recommends that patients with advanced cancer should receive dedicated palliative care services, within eight weeks of diagnosis concurrent with active treatment. Providers may refer caregivers of patients with early or advanced cancer to palliative care services. For palliative care in Malaysia, the CPG for Breast Cancer Management (2010) recommends that palliative care physician should be involved in the management of advanced breast cancer.

2.5 UHC in Cancer

During the conduct of this study, a consolidated research on UHC of cancer in Malaysia was not yet available. However, there were two major studies which explored the components of UHC of cancer such as quality of care, accessibility, effective coverage and out-of-pocket expenditure.

2.5.1 Service coverage

One landmark local multi-center, retrospective observational cohort study which investigated the service accessibility and performance for breast cancer treatment was carried out by Lim et al. (2014) among 750 breast cancer patients in eight hospitals in Malaysia. In that study, performance of breast cancer care was assessed using measures developed by Quality Oncology Practice Initiative (QOPI), American Society of Clinical Oncology/ National Comprehensive Cancer Network (ASCO/NCCN), American College of Surgeons' National Accreditation Program for Breast Centers, and the Malaysian CPG on Breast Cancer Management.

Results from this study indicated that access to diagnostic and breast surgery services was generally good where 70% to 82% of cases adhered to the performance measures for surgery, chemotherapy, radiation therapy and hormonal therapy. Adherence meant that the patients received the required treatment in the specified timeframe. However, this study reported that access to targeted therapy with the drug Trastuzumab, was limited to only 19% of eligible patients. According to the researchers, the inaccessibility to this population to Trastuzumab was believed to be due to absence of public funding support. The researchers concluded that these performance results were probably acceptable for a middle-income country. This study was significant because it had indirectly measured effective coverage of the entire treatment course of breast cancer. However, the study did not address financial protection coverage.

2.5.2 Financial protection coverage

Financial protection coverage was addressed in another study called the ACTION (Asean CosTs In Oncology) study (ACTION Study Group 2015). The ACTION study was a prospective, multinational study. Results from the study showed that the majority of low- and middle-income countries (LMICs) in the ASEAN region did not have universal health coverage; hence patients experienced high out-of-pocket expenses which led to financial catastrophe and economic hardship. The study also found that at the end of one year following diagnosis, 48% of the cancer patient experienced financial catastrophe (defined as spending on health care more than 30% of household income) and 29% had died (ACTION Study Group 2015). A third of those (33%) who had no economic hardship at baseline experienced economic hardship at one year, of whom 45% were unable to pay for medicines (Bhoo-Pathy 2015).

2.6 Conceptual Framework

The general objective of this study was to determine the extent of universal health coverage in breast cancer management in Malaysia. From the available literature discussed earlier, the conceptual framework in Figure 2.9 was developed. This framework also served as the UHC monitoring framework for this study.

The framework focuses on two main determinants of UHC, which are service coverage and financial protection coverage. Service coverage has two part: service coverage for prevention measures and service coverage for treatment measures. The service coverage part in the framework was adapted from the framework proposed by Boerma et al. (2014).

Financial protection coverage is determined by the catastrophic health expenditure and impoverishment among patients who received treatment for breast cancer, adapted from the Global Monitoring Report (WHO 2015). Socioeconomic factors can influence the prevalence of catastrophic health expenditure and impoverishment and thus included in this framework.

The building blocks of the health system become the foundation for the framework in achieving UHC. The entire UHC framework rests on this foundation. These building blocks are adapted from the handbook of indicators and measurements to monitor the building blocks of health system (WHO 2010b). As mentioned in available literature discussed earlier, these building blocks, sometimes referred to as input and output factors, do not directly contribute in determining the UHC index, but they help to explain the UHC index score by putting the score into context.

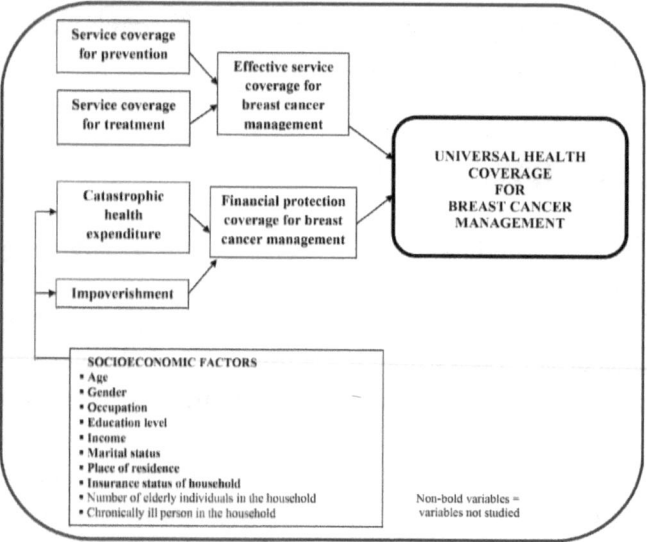

Figure 2.9 Conceptual framework for UHC monitoring

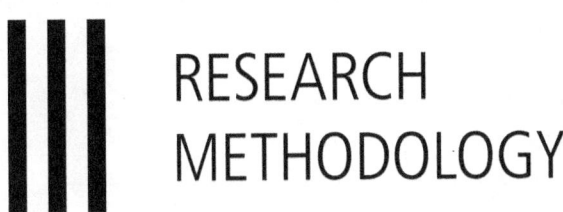
RESEARCH METHODOLOGY

3.1 Introduction

This study aimed to assess the extent of universal health coverage (UHC) in breast cancer management in Malaysia. This study comprised of two components, two parts and two segments.

Component 1 addressed the first research objective, which was to develop the framework, indicators and targets for assessing the extent of UHC of breast cancer management in Malaysia from the currently available criteria and indicators. In Component 2, assessment of variables of UHC was done based on the indicators and targets. Component 2 were further divided into two parts: Part 1 and Part 2.

Part 1 was to address the second research objective, which was: to determine if the building blocks of the Malaysian health system are available, including that for breast cancer management. Part 1 involved data collection on the availability of building blocks of the health system through database and reports review. Part 2 was to address the third through sixth research objectives, which were: to determine the extent of effective service coverage in breast cancer management, to determine the extent of financial protection coverage among breast cancer patients and their households, to determine the associating and predicting factors of catastrophic health expenditure and impoverishment among breast cancer patients and their households, and to calculate the composite index score of UHC in breast cancer management. Part 2 were further divided into two segments: Segment 1 (Service Coverage) and Segment 2 (Financial Protection Coverage). The study framework is as shown in Figure 3.1.

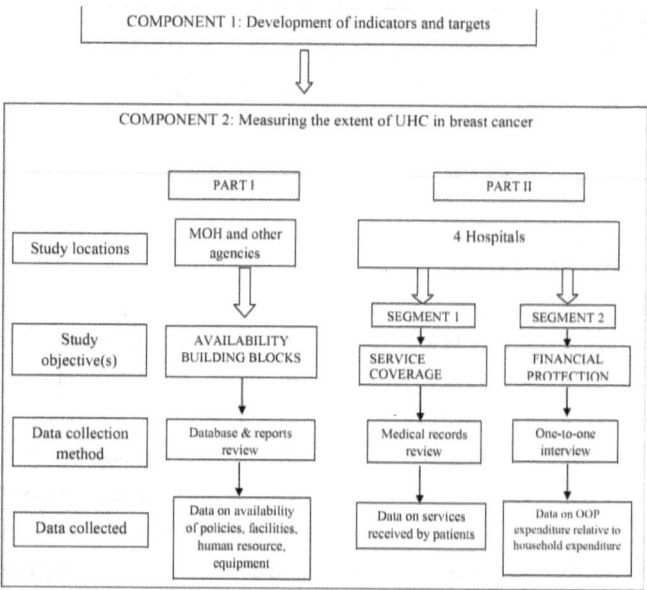

Figure 3.1 Study framework

3.2 Component 1: Development of indicators and targets

Component 1 of the study aimed to address the first study objective which was to develop the framework, indicators and targets for the UHC monitoring for breast cancer management in Malaysia.

3.2.1 The compilation of service coverage indicator criteria

The framework to assess the extent of UHC in breast cancer management was presented earlier as the conceptual framework of this study. The next step was to compile indicator criteria before coming up with the indictors.

Literature review was conducted to find the criteria for the indicators of UHC monitoring. Three major sources of UHC indicator criteria were found. The first was the Bellagio Centre of the Rockefeller Foundation Report produced in September 2012. This report suggested the use of tracer indicators (Rockefeller Foundation Center Bellagio 2012). Criteria of these tracer indicators were: 1) of high epidemiological relevance, 2) have evidence-based intervention that is effective, 3) measureable for both numerator and denominator with minimal reliance to modelling for the denominator, 4) its results should be easy to understand and communicate, and 5) universality or being relevant in many settings. Additionally, the report suggested that an indicator or index was more meaningful if clear targets were set. Ideally such targets, with an annual rate of progress and target year, would be based on historical data from best performing countries. For the dimensions of health service coverage, the goal would be to achieve complete coverage (100%) for key interventions, or in the shorter run rates above 80% or 90% in all population strata. In this report, the quality of care dimension was also proposed. Three methods were suggested: 1) using effective coverage (defined as the fraction of maximum possible health gain an individual with a health care need can expect to receive from the health system), 2) using readily available quality of care indicators such as those of OECD's indicators which linked quality of health services and health system performance. The indicators ranged from health impacts (e.g. five-year survival rates for different cancers), to outcomes (e.g. coverage with a set of key preventive services such as mammography screening) to outputs (avoidable hospital admissions for asthma), covering selected tracer areas: cancer care, mental health, prevention and promotion, patient safety and patient experience, and 3) to use availability and readiness indices. For instance, the availability of tracer drugs which were the WHO fourteen generic drugs. If the drugs were present it did not guarantee good quality of care, but if they were not available good quality of care was not likely. In terms of financial hardship this meeting proposed the impoverishment indicator and the extent of OOP expenditure for health.

The second was the WHO and WBG document published in 2014, which recommended the adoption of a small set of indicators to track progress was as there were many service coverage indicators (WHO 2014a). The "tracer" indicators were to follow these criteria: 1) relevance, 2) quality and 3) availability of data. UHC indicators should include both prevention and treatment coverage. The core set of interventions could be built over time as and when comparable, reliable measures of coverage for other intervention areas, such as rehabilitation and palliation, become available. Like the earlier discussion paper, financial protection coverage uses the two commonly used indicators: incidence of "catastrophic" health expenditures and the incidence of impoverishment due to out-of-pocket health payments. This document also introduced the use of equity measurement: three primary elements for disaggregation that can be measured comparably in all settings were proposed. These were: 1) household income, expenditure or wealth (coverage of the poorest segment of the population as compared with richer segments), 2) place of residence (rural or urban) and 3) gender. Lastly for targets, this document proposed the ultimate target was 100% coverage. For some services, such as treatment of hypertension, effective coverage can reach 100% only if the treatment is 100% effective, which is rarely the case. Likewise, treatment indicators (such as for HIV infection) are often based on estimated need, which is rarely sufficiently accurate to set a target of 100%.

The third was an article published in 2014 based on the technical meeting of principal investigators of UHC organized by the WHO and Ministry of Health of Singapore held in Singapore in September 2013 (Boerma et al 2014). The proposed criteria for UHC monitoring indicators were similar to the preceding list but were more detailed: 1) the indicator should measure an intervention associated with a significant proportion of the potential burden of disease, 2) the indicator must be evidence-based and showed that the intervention which the indicator measured was effective and feasible to deliver, 3) both numerator (the population receiving the intervention) and denominator (the population needing the intervention) of the coverage indicator should be well defined, 4) that the ultimate target for all indicators was 100%, 5) indicator disaggregation should be possible by age, household wealth/income, gender, residence (urban/rural, province, district), ethnicity, and other key stratifiers, 6) the intervention needed to be delivered with the level of quality necessary to achieve the desired outcome, 7) all indicators needed to be measurable in a comparable way over time and across countries, 8) indicators must be easy to convey to policy makers and the general public, 9) availability of quality comparable coverage data should be ensured, 10) extent to which indicators have been recommended (and used) in international initiatives should be considered, such as the MDGs and 11) the number of tracer indicators should be kept small. Based on these sources, a list of UHC service coverage indicator criteria were compiled as summarized in Table 3.1, while the criteria for effective service coverage as detailed by Ng at al. (2014) are listed in Table 3.2.

Table 3.1 UHC service coverage indicator criteria

Criteria for indicators	Source of indicator
1. Condition is of high epidemiological relevance	Rockefeller Foundation Center Bellagio (2012); WHO (2014a); Boerma et al. (2014)
2. Have evidence-based intervention that is effective	Rockefeller Foundation Center Bellagio (2012); Boerma et al. (2014)
3. Measurable for both numerator and denominator	Rockefeller Foundation Center Bellagio (2012); Boerma et al. (2014)
4. Numerators and denominators are well-defined	Boerma et al. (2014)
5. Services which are cost-effective	WHO (2014a)
6. Service coverage which are effective or quality-adjusted	WHO (2014a), Boerma et al. (2014)
7. The interventions chosen, have potential financial risks to user/ involves major health expenditure	WHO (2014a)
8. Ultimate target for indicators is set at 100%	Boerma et al. (2014)
9. Disaggregation by social stratifiers such as age, ethnicity	Rockefeller Foundation Center Bellagio (2012); Boerma et al. (2014)
10. Have readily available data	WHO (2014a); Boerma et al. (2014)
11. Results easy to understand, communicate	Rockefeller Foundation Center Bellagio (2012); Boerma et al. (2014)
12. Universality/ relevant in many settings	Rockefeller Foundation Center Bellagio (2012);
13. Comparable over time and in many countries	Boerma et al. (2014)
14. Part of international initiatives	Boerma et al. (2014)
15. The number of indicators should be kept small.	Boerma et al. (2014)

Table 3.2 Effective coverage metrics

Effective coverage metrics	Explanation
1. Need	The measure of intervention need is whether an individual would benefit from receiving a specific health intervention.
2. Use	Intervention use reflects whether an individual, conditional on needing the intervention, received or used a specific intervention.
3. Quality	Intervention quality captures whether a specific intervention conferred the health gain or protection it was supposed to (effectiveness).

Next, the list of relevant indicators for UHC service coverage of breast cancer management for this study was constructed. This current study proposed the use suitable quality performance indicators (QPIs) as these service coverage indicators.

3.2.2 The rationale of using quality performance indicators (QPI) as service coverage indicators

During the literature review process, it was noted that most quality performance indicators (QPIs) used in the clinical setting seemed to fulfill the criteria of the UHC service indicators. QPIs in the clinical setting were often described as the percentage of patients who received the care they need within a specified timeframe. For example, one QPI from the American College of Surgeons-National Comprehensive Cancer Network (ASCO-NCCN) reads: "Adjuvant multi-agent (combination) chemotherapy for women under age 70 with Stage I (Tc) to III ER/PR negative breast cancer within 120 days of date of diagnosis" (ASCO-NCCN Quality Measures for Breast and Colorectal Cancer Care).

The QPI stated above fulfilled 12 of the 14 of the criteria for UHC monitoring indicators. The two criteria not fulfilled were 1) the service target set at 100%, which was not possible for treatment for breast cancer in general, and 2) able to measure equity which shall be addressed by the financial protection indicator. The adherence of the abovementioned QPI to the criteria for UHC monitoring indicators is shown in Table 3.3.

Table 3.3 Adherence of QPI to the criteria for UHC monitoring indicators

Criteria for indicators	Adherence
1. Condition is of high epidemiological relevance	Yes
2. Have evidence-based intervention that is effective	Yes
3. Measurable for both numerator and denominator	Yes
4. Numerators and denominators are well-defined	Yes
5. Services which are cost-effective	Yes
6. Service coverage which are effective or quality-adjusted	Yes
7. The interventions chosen, have potential financial risks to user/involves major health expenditure	Yes
8. Ultimate target for indicators is set at 100%	Not possible
9. Disaggregation by social stratifiers such as age, ethnicity	Possible
10. Have readily available data	Yes
11. Results easy to understand, communicate	Yes
12. Universality/ relevant in many settings	Yes
13. Comparable over time and in many countries	Yes
14. Part of international initiatives	Yes
15. The number of indicators should be kept small.	Yes

Additionally, these indicators fulfilled the criteria for effective coverage, which were - 1) need (the need for the intervention), 2) use (the utilization of the intervention) and 3) quality (the quality of the intervention). Hence for the same QPI mentioned above, its adherence to the criteria for effective service coverage is detailed in Table 3.4.

Table 3.4 Adherence to the criteria for effective service coverage

Criteria for effective service coverage	Adherence
1. Need	Need was specified in the abovementioned indicator which was "women under the age of 70 with Stage I (Tc) to III ER/PR negative breast cancer". A woman who fits this criterion would benefit from this intervention, as evidenced by currently available clinical evidence.
2. Use	Use was captured by this indicator because the study determined the number of patients who received this intervention.
3. Quality	Quality in is embedded in the indicator, where the indicator had specified the treatment (adjuvant multi-agent (combination) chemotherapy), the type of patient who would most benefit from it (women under the age of 70 with Stage I (Tc) to III ER/PR negative breast cancer) and the time frame the intervention need to be given to give the best outcome (within 120 days of date of diagnosis).

Based on this finding, other QPIs on breast cancer management were searched to ultimately produce a set of indicators for UHC effective service coverage of breast cancer management. The steps involved are discussed in the following section. Lastly, by adopting the currently available financial protection coverage indicators, a comprehensive set of UHC monitoring indicators for breast cancer management was formed.

3.2.3 Steps in developing the proposed indicators for UHC in breast cancer management

The steps involved in the development of the indicators were as follows. Firstly, for service coverage for UHC of breast cancer, online search for QPIs on breast cancer management were carried out. Keywords used were a combination of "quality performance indicators", "quality indicators", "process indicators", "effective service coverage",

"QPI" and "breast cancer" with the following components of breast cancer management: "screening", "mammogram", "chemotherapy", "radiotherapy", "neoadjuvant chemotherapy", "mastectomy", "breast conservation surgery", "endocrine therapy", "hormone therapy", "targeted therapy", "palliative care" and "morphine".

The inclusion criteria for the search were literature in the English language and published between the year 2010 and 2015. The exclusion criteria for the search were outcome indicators of breast cancer management and general indicators such as indicators related to the health systems.

Process indicators were selected and not outcome indicators, because even though clinical outcome measures are the gold standard for measuring effectiveness in health care, they are potentially be problematic to be assessed, especially in the case of cancer as the outcomes cannot realistically be determined in a timely or feasible fashion. Process indicators were also selected because they were used in the first global report on UHC monitoring and their uses for cervical cancer screening were discussed in the Meeting on Monitoring Universal Health Coverage in Rockefeller Centre in November 2015 (WHO 2015).

Once the search for effective service coverage was completed, the search for financial protection coverage was carried out. Financial protection coverage indicators were noted to be generic in nature and can be used in any nature of diseases or illness.

Lastly, already available indicators for the building blocks for the health system were compiled. These indicators were also generic in nature and can be used in any nature of diseases or illness.

3.2.4 Proposed indicators for UHC in breast cancer management

a. Proposed indicator the UHC monitoring of breast cancer

For prevention coverage, the QPI selected was mammogram screening uptake. According to the Malaysian CPG on

Breast Cancer Management (2010), breast cancer screening is recommended among women aged 50-74 years, but women aged 40-49 years may undergo the mammogram screening if they wish.

As for treatment coverage Greenberg et al. (2005) had summarized several organizations around the world which have developed comprehensive performance measurement systems, as shown in Table 3.5. Several of the quality assessment tools are discussed in the following paragraphs, as well as those of NICE (UK) and Malaysia.

Table 3.5 Organizations with performance measurement systems

	Organization	Cancers	Services	Region
1.	European Cancer Health Indicator Project (EUROCHIP)	All	Prevention, screening, treatment, palliation	European Union
2.	American Society of Clinical Oncology (ASCO)	Breast, colon/rectum	Diagnosis, treatment	United States of America (five cities)
3.	National Cancer Institute (NCI)	Breast, cervix, colorectal, all sites combined	Prevention, early detection, diagnosis, follow-up, end-of-life	US national
4.	RAND Corporation	Breast, cervical, colorectal, lung, prostate, skin	Screening, diagnosis, treatment, follow-up/ palliation	US National
5.	National Health Service (NHS)	Breast, colorectal, lung	Prevention, early detection, treatment, palliation	UK national
6.	National Comprehensive Cancer Network (NCCN)	Breast, non-Hodgkin's lymphoma	Treatment, pain assessment and management	US NCCN member cancer centers

The main contributor for breast cancer quality or performance measures was the United States of America (USA) where efforts in the development of quality performance measures for cancer began in the year 1999 (Malin et al. 2006). In the year 2000 the

American Society of Clinical Oncologists (ASCO) conducted the first ever comprehensive, multicenter study called the National Initiative for Cancer Care Quality (NICCQ), following reports which claimed that cancer patients were not receiving optimal care (Malin et al. 2006). In this NICCQ study, 36 quality and performance indicators were developed (Appendix A5).

In 2007 and 2008 ASCO collaborated with the National Comprehensive Cancer Network (NCCN) to develop a set of measures for breast and colorectal cancers based on the NICCQ quality measures. ASCO and NCCN also used the method by Hasset et al. (2008) in determining the quality indicator selection (Albert & Das 2010). Based on data from the NICCQ and NCCN measures, the ASCO/NCCN panels recommended three measures for breast cancer and four measures for colorectal cancer. The developed measures were subsequently synchronized with similar measures developed by the Commission of Cancer (CoC) of the American College of Surgeons (ACoS). The final measures for breast cancer are shown in Table 3.6 (Desch et al. 2008).

Table 3.6 Final Measures as Harmonized by ASCO/NCCN and CoC and Endorsed by the National Quality Forum

Breast cancer treatment	Indicators
Surgery	Not available
Chemotherapy	Adjuvant multi-agent (combination) chemotherapy for women under age 70 with Stage I (Tc) to III ER/PR negative breast cancer within 120 days of date of diagnosis.
Radiation therapy	Radiation therapy for women under age 70 with Stage I to III breast cancer who had breast conserving surgery for breast cancer within 1 year (365 days) of date of diagnosis.
Hormone therapy	Tamoxifen or Aromatase Inhibitor for women greater than age 17 with Stage I to III ER or PR positive breast cancer within 1 year (365 days) of date of diagnosis.
Targeted therapy	Not available
Palliative care	Not available

Over the years, these breast cancer quality measures from the NCCN and ASCO have been adopted in several studies, both within the USA and globally. For example, they were used in the Florida Initiative for Quality Cancer Care (FIQCC) study (Laronga et al. 2014); in breast cancer quality assessment among vulnerable population in the US (Chen et al. 2011); in the development a new set of quality indicators in China (Bao et al. 2015) and to measure the performance of breast cancer management in Malaysia by Lim et al. (2014).

In the US, apart from ASCO-NCCN-ACoS, the National Cancer Institute in the United States has two quality indicators for breast cancer which were: 1) Percentage of women aged 20 and older, diagnosed with early stage breast cancer (less than stage IIIA), receiving breast-conserving surgery and radiation treatment, and 2) Percentage of women aged 20 and older, diagnosed with node-positive, stage I–IIIA breast cancer, receiving multi-agent chemotherapy.

In Europe, the National Institute for Health and Care Excellence (NICE) of the National Health Service (NHS) United Kingdom (UK) has a quality standard for breast cancer developed in 2011 and has been recently improved in 2016. The NICE quality standard consists of six quality statements (Appendix A6). Apart from NICE, the European Society of Breast Cancer Specialists (EUSOMA) had also produced a set of QPIs consisting of 17 indicators in 2010 and revised in 2014 (Appendix A7).

In Malaysia, the Malaysian CPG for breast cancer management (2010) proposed three clinical audit indicators for quality management: on initial treatment, post-surgery chemotherapy and local recurrence. More recently, based on the National Strategic Plan for Cancer Control Program 2016-2020 there are two indicators to measure the performance of breast cancer management: on waiting time to get an appointment for referral and on waiting time for surgery (Ministry of Health 2016a).

Table 3.7 Quality performance indicators for breast cancer, Malaysia

Breast cancer treatment	MOH Malaysia indicators
1. Surgery	• Percentage of newly diagnosed breast cancer patients receiving initial treatment within two months of presentation
2. Chemotherapy	• Percentage of eligible breast cancer patients' post-surgery commencing chemotherapy within two months. • Percentage of patients going for definitive surgery for breast cancer within 4 weeks of the diagnosis. The target was set at >75%
3. Radiation therapy	• Not available
4. Hormone therapy	• Not available
5. Targeted therapy	• Not available
6. Palliative care	• Not available
7. Others	• Percentage of local recurrence of breast cancer within two years • Percentage of patients given appointment at Breast Clinic for a suspicious breast lump/lesion within 14 working days of referral. The target was set at > 80%

The indicators from these major sources provide indicators for most of the treatment components of breast cancer: surgery, chemotherapy and part of radiotherapy. However, even though the quality measurement indicators of the NICCQ was the most comprehensive and comprised of 36 indicators, they did not have indicators on radiation therapy. The ASCO-NCCN indicators however only had indicator for radiation therapy among patients who had undergone lumpectomy, while indicator for radiation therapy for women who had undergone mastectomy was available from the Commission on Cancer (CoC) of the American College of Surgeons. As for targeted therapy, only ASCO had the quality indicator for the use of the drug Trastuzmab.

As for palliative care, none of these sets of indicators had any indicator on palliative care. However, the World Health Organization Global Monitoring Framework on non-communicable diseases has the indicator for the service coverage for palliative care. In 2012 this indicator was stated as "access to palliative care assessed by morphine equivalent consumption of strong opioid analgesics (excluding methadone & pethidine) per capita". This indicator was later changed in 2015 to "Indicator 20 - Access to palliative care assessed by morphine-equivalent consumption of strong opioid analgesics (excluding methadone) per death from cancer" (WHO 2013b).

Table 3.8 Quality performance indicators for palliative care

Breast cancer treatment	WHO Global Monitoring Framework in NCDs indicator on palliative care
a. Surgery	Not available
b. Chemotherapy	Not available
c. Radiation therapy	Not available
d. Hormone therapy	Not available
e. Targeted therapy	Not available
f. Palliative care	Access to palliative care assessed by morphine-equivalent consumption of strong opioid analgesics (excluding methadone) per death from cancer

The summary of the quality performance indicators for palliative care is as shown in the following Table 3.9.

Table 3.9 Quality performance indicators for palliative care

Treatment option	Indicator	Numerator (Number of patients who obtained the treatment option)	Denominator (Number of patients eligible for inclusion for the treatment option)	Result (Percent of patients whose care adhere with treatment option)
Screening	Woman 40 - 74 years old who undergone mammogram			
Surgery	Patients under age 70 with Stage I to III Breast cancer who received surgery within 2 months of diagnosis			
Chemotherapy	Adjuvant multi-agent (combination) chemotherapy for women under age 70 with Stage I (Tc) to III ER/PR negative breast cancer within 120 days of date of diagnosis			
Radiation therapy	Radiation therapy for women under age 70 with Stage I to III breast cancer who had breast conserving surgery (BCS) for breast cancer within 1 year (365 days) of date of diagnosis Radiation therapy for women under age 70 who had mastectomy for breast cancer with node+ (four or more positive regional lymph nodes) within 1 year (365 days) of date of diagnosis			
Hormonal therapy	Tamoxifen or Aromatase Inhibitor for women greater than age 17 with Stage I to III ER or PR positive breast cancer within 1 year (365 days) of date of diagnosis			
Targeted therapy	Trastuzumab therapy for women greater than age 17 with Stage I (Tc) to III HER2 positive breast cancer			
Palliative care	Access to palliative care assessed by morphine-equivalent consumption of strong opioid analgesics (excluding methadone) per death from cancer			

b. Proposed indicators for building blocks of the health system

As health system strengthening is essential for the achievement of universal health coverage, these building blocks of the health system were included in this study. In the Donabedian-based UHC monitoring framework by Boerma et al (2014), the inputs and outputs in that framework correspond to these building blocks of the health system. The WHO (2010) proposed 10 indicators to monitor leadership and governance in health. This set of indicators is called the Policy Index. For breast cancer, five of these indicators are relevant to breast cancer management (indicators 1, 2, 3, 9, 10).

As health system strengthening is essential for the achievement of universal health coverage, these building blocks of the health system were included in this study. In the Donabedian-based UHC monitoring framework by Boerma et al. (2014), the inputs and outputs in that framework correspond to these building blocks of the health system.

The WHO in its guidebook, proposed the following indicators for the building blocks of the health system (WHO 2010b). There are ten indicators to monitor leadership and governance in health. This set of indicators is called the Policy Index. For breast cancer, five of these indicators are relevant to breast cancer management which were Indicators 1, 2, 3, 9, 10 (Appendix A8). There are three core indicators for health systems financing. Although these indicators are not cancer-specific they do give an overview of the current financing situation of the health service which influences cancer management (Appendix A9). Additionally, there are 30 indicators proposed by the WHO for health information system, but there are no indicators specifically to assess health information system for cancer (Appendix A10).

The current literature however has shown that in terms of health information system in cancer care, the focus has been on the use of geographical information system (Fradelos et al. 2014; Mechili et al. 2014; Musa et al. 2013), electronic health records for cancer patients (Fasola et al. 2014), personalized hospital information system (HIS) for cancer patients (Clauser et al. 2011) and the development of registries namely clinic, laboratory and referral registries. For access to medicine are five proposed indicators (Appendix A11). Although these indicators were not cancer-specific they do give an overview of the current access to essential medicines and its effects on cancer management (WHO 2010b). In terms of cancer treatment, the list of essential medicines for cancer was obtained from the WHO source (Robertson et al.2016) (Appendix A12).

The indicators for service-specific availability are available from the WHO's Service Availability and Readiness Assessment (SARA) module (WHO 2013c). Service availability is concerned with the physical presence of items required for the delivery of services and encompasses 1) health infrastructure (number and distribution of health facilities), 2) health workforce of core health personnel (number and distribution of core medical professionals per 10,000 populations) and 3) service utilization (Appendices A13 and A14).

Lastly, the targets for these indicators were determined. The available targets for the indicators are listed in Table 3.10. For the other indicators, there were no specific targets, instead those indicators were meant to be used as dashboard monitoring of the progress of the indicators over the years.

Table 3.10 Targets for UHC indicators

Indicator	Coverage	Source
1. Screening	70%	WHO
2. Treatment	80%	WHO
3. Palliative care	100%	WHO
4. TEH from GDP	5-6%	WBG
5. GHE from GGE	8%	WBG
6. OOPE from TEH	15-20%.	WBG

3.3 Component 2: Measuring the extent of UHC in breast cancer

3.3.1 Part 1: Determine the availability of building blocks for UHC

Part 1 of the study was to answer the first study objective, namely, to determine the availability of the building blocks for UHC in breast cancer management. In the conceptual framework these refer to the input and output factors. If these factors were not available, the country's ability to attain universal health coverage may be reduced.

a. Objective

The objective of this part of the study was to describe the availability of the building blocks of services in breast cancer management.

b. Data collection method

Most of the information required for this part of the study was obtained from published documents, web-based sources, cancer registries, project reports, and interviews with those responsible for cancer-related matters at the country level. Publicly available official reports and websites of private entities relevant to this study were also reviewed.

To determine service-specific readiness, the ability of health facilities to offer a specific service, and the capacity to provide that service, were measured through the following domains: 1) trained staff, 2) equipment, 3) diagnostic capacity and 4) medicines and commodities. Each domain consists of a set of tracer items. These indicators were as shown in Table 3.11 using mammogram service as an example. As shown in Table 3.11, for each service, the number of facilities with the tracer indicators ("a", "p" and "s") was then divided total number of facilities ("b", "q" and "t"), to get the proportion ("c", "r" and "u"). The proportion was divided by the number of tracer indicators to get the mean domain score ("A" and "B"). Each mean domain score was summed and divided by the total number of tracer indicators for the service (involving all the domains), to get the sum of domain score ("z"). This sum of domain score was then multiplied by 100% to get the percentage domain score.

Table 3.11 Service readiness for breast cancer management

Service	Domain	Tracer indicator	Proportion of facilities with the tracer indicator †	Mean domain score	Sum availability/ no. of tracer indicators	Percentage domain score
Mammogram	Trained staff, Guidelines	Radiographer	a/b = c	[c+r+u]/3 = A	[A+ B]/4 = z	z x 100%
		Radiologist	p/q = r			
		CPGs, SOPs	s/t = u			
Equipment		Mammogram machines	u/v = w	w/1 = B		
Surgery	Trained staff	General surgeons, breast surgeons				
	Guidelines	CPGs, SOPs				
	Equipment	General operating theatre				
Chemotherapy	Trained staff	Clinical oncologist				
		Oncology trained nurses				
		CDR pharmacist				
	Guidelines, Equipment	CPGs, SOPs				
		CDR pharmacy, clean room				
Radiotherapy	Trained staff	Physicist				
	Guidelines	CPGs, SOPs				
	Equipment	Megavoltage machines				

Note: † = number of facilities offering the service (example: mammogram) which had the tracer indicator, divided by the total number of facilities offering the service (example: mammogram).

3.3.2 Part 2: Determine the effective service coverage and the financial protection coverage.

a. Objective

Part 2 of the study aimed to address the third and fourth research objectives: to determine the effective service coverage and the financial protection coverage. Therefore Part 2 of this study was further divided into two segments: Segment 1 and Segment 2. Data collection in Segment I was to address effective service coverage, while data collection in Segment II was to address financial protection coverage. Data collected from Segment I and Segment II were also subsequently jointly analyzed to address the fifth and sixth objectives: to determine factors associated with catastrophic health expenditure and impoverishment among breast cancer patients and to calculate the composite index score of UHC in breast cancer management.

b. Study location

The study was carried out in four referral tertiary level hospitals with surgical, oncology and radiation therapy services (Hospital Kuala Lumpur, Hospital Putrajaya and National Cancer Institute; as well as Hospital Canselor Tuanku Muhriz/Universiti Kebangsaan Malaysia Medical Centre). These were referral hospitals located in the west coast and central region of Peninsula Malaysia.

c. Study duration

This study was from 2015 to 2017.

d. **Study population**

The study population was female breast cancer patients, who came to the study sites for breast cancer treatment between January 2015 and January 2017.

e. **Sampling unit**

The sampling unit was one breast cancer patient.

f. **Sample size**

For Segment I (service coverage), the minimum sample size was also calculated using a formula for prevalence studies (Lwanga and Lemeshow, 1991), as follows.

Sample size (n) = [($z_{1-\alpha}$)2 * p(1-p)] ÷ d2
where: $z_{1-\alpha}$ = 1.96, d = 0.05, p = population proportion.

For service coverage, the prevalence values were based on the study by Lim et al. (2014) on breast cancer performance measures, as detailed in Table 3.12. The sampling unit was the medical record of one breast cancer patient. The minimum sample size required was set at 288.

Table 3.12 Sample size options for service coverage

Performance measures for cancer treatment services	p = proportion	Sample size
1. Patients under age 70 with Stage I to III Breast cancer who received Surgery within 2 months of diagnosis	0.82	228
2. Adjuvant multi-agent (combination) chemotherapy for women under age 70 with Stage I (Tc) to III ER/PR negative breast cancer within 120 days of date of diagnosis	0.75	288
3. Radiation therapy for women under age 70 with Stage I to III breast cancer who had breast conserving surgery for breast cancer within 1 year (365 days) of date of diagnosis	0.77	272
4. Radiation therapy for women under age 70 who had mastectomy for breast cancer with node+ (four or more positive regional lymph nodes) within 1 year (365 days) of date of diagnosis	0.81	236
5. Tamoxifen or Aromatase Inhibitor for women greater than age 17 with Stage I to III ER or PR positive breast cancer within 1 year (365 days) of date of diagnosis	0.76	280
6. Trastuzumab therapy for women greater than age 17 with Stage I (Tc) to III HER2 positive breast cancer within 1 year (365 days) of date of diagnosis	0.19	236

For Segment II (financial protection coverage), the calculations were based on one proportion and two proportions formula accordingly to satisfy the objectives and variables of the study. The sample size was estimated using multiple references.

The minimum sample size required for the prevalence of catastrophic health expenditure was calculated using the formula for proportion studies (Lwanga & Lemeshow 1991).

Sample size (n) = [(z 1-α)2 * p(1-p)] ÷ d2
where:
z1-α = standard normal variate at 5% type 1 error, p < 0.05; hence = 1.96
d = absolute error or precision = 0.05
p = proportion in population based on previous studies

The minimum sample size required for the comparison between two groups was calculated using the formula for two proportion studies (Lwanga & Lemeshow 1991).

Sample size (n) = (z α/2 + z β)2 * p1(1-p1) + p2(1-p2)] ÷ [(p1 - p2)2]
where:
z α/2 = standard normal variate of type 1 error, at 5% error, p < 0.05; hence, z α/2 =1.96
z β = standard normal variate of power; at 80% power hence, z β = 0.84
p1 = proportion in population with CHE with risk factor based on previous studies
p2 = proportion in population with CHE without risk factor based on previous studies

At present, there are several studies on catastrophic health expenditure in Malaysia and the ASEAN region. The landmark study on health expenditure among cancer patients entitled Asean CosTs In ONcology (ACTION study), showed that the proportion of cancer patients (all cancer types) who suffered from CHE was 48 %. For breast cancer patients, the proportion of them who suffered CHE was approximately 60%. In a study in South Korea among cancer patients, the results showed that the proportion of patients with CHE was 39.8% (Cho et al. 2014). In a local study, the proportion of CHE in Malaysia was between 0.3% and 1.1% (Ng 2015); while in the 2002/03 World Health Survey household-level data from four Asia Pacific countries (China, Malaysia, Philippines and Vietnam), the proportion was 4.6% (Reddy et al. 2013).

For catastrophic health expenditure, the minimum sample size was calculated using the prevalence formula (Lwanga & Lemeshaw, 1991), based on the prevalence of CHE from several studies. For factors associated with CHE, the minimum sample size was calculated using the 2-proportions formula (Lwanga & Lemeshaw, 1991). The $z_{1-\alpha}$ = 1.96, d = 0.05, p = population proportion.

Table 3.13 Sample size options for financial coverage

Study variable	Study	Proportion of CHE	Sample size
Prevalence of CHE	ACTION study (2015)	All cancers 48%,	384
		Breast cancer 60% (At threshold of equal to or exceeding 30 % of annual household income)	368
Prevalence of CHE	Choi et al. (2014)	39.8%	368
Chronic illness	Van Minh et al. (2012)	P1 = 7.6% (no chronic illness) P2 = 2.3% (with chronic illnes)	204
Household income	Delavari et al. (2014)	P1 = 67.5% (low income) P2 = 75.0% (high income)	649
Family size	Delavari et al. (2014)	P1 = 28.2% (small family) P2 = 19.6% (large family)	444

For the minimum sample size required for impoverishment due to health expenditure was calculated using a formula for proportion studies *(Lwanga and Lemeshow 1991)*, where: $z_{1-\alpha}$ = 1.96, d = 0.05, p = population proportion. As the proportion of impoverishment in health expenditure for cancer was not available during the time of the study, the proportion value used was 0.5.

Sample size (n) = [(z 1-α)2 * p(1-p)] ÷ d2
= 384

With the non-response rate of approximately 2% as detected during the pilot study, the number of respondents to be sampled was set at 390. The number of respondents was sampled proportionally to the number of beds at the oncology day care facility of the study sites.

g. Sampling method

In Segment I, where effective service coverage was determined, the data collection was done retrospectively. Prospective data collection was not practical due to time and resource constraints. Additionally, there may be crossover of patients between the private and the public hospitals (Lim et al. 2014). Therefore, retrospective data collection was a more suitable approach in this study because the study sites were government hospitals.

A list of patients who attended the oncology clinic and day care chemotherapy services between 2015 and 2016 was used as the sampling frame. Name of each patient was given a number in ascending order. The list of numbers was then imputed into a computer software to choose random numbers. The numbers generated by the software was then matched with the patient name list and the corresponding patients then retrieved. Cases which fulfilled the inclusion criteria were included in the study. The inclusion criteria were Malaysian female breast cancer cases, in stage I, II or III, and diagnosed not earlier than 2013. Cases which did not meet these criteria were excluded from the study. Resampling was done to the remaining cases in the list and the screening process was repeated until the required sample size (290 cases) was obtained.

For Segment II, purposive sampling method was used. Patients who attended the clinic and oncology day care between 2016 and 2017, and who fulfilled the inclusion criteria were invited to participate in the study. Inclusion criteria for were female patients treated for breast cancer, Malaysian citizen aged more than 18 years old, at any stage of breast cancer, has been receiving active treatment in the last one year, not clinically ill and was comfortable to answer questions

h. Data collection method

For Segment I, the data were collected by the reviewing the medical records of cases which fulfilled the inclusion criteria. Only four types of data were collected: 1) date of birth, 2) TNM staging, 3) biomarker status (ER/PR/HER2), and 4) the starting dates of the breast cancer treatment/interventions. No personal identification data was collected.

For Segment II, names of breast cancer patients at the oncology clinic and day care unit were identified from the patient name list or register available at the premises on the day of data collection. These breast cancer patients were approached. Those who fulfilled the inclusion criteria were informed about the study, the study objectives and what was required from them. After obtaining consent from the respondent, data was collected one-to-one using a data collection form by the researcher collection tool.

i. Data collection tool

The data collection tool for Segment 1 was a data collection form. The form contained the following required data: 1) date of birth, 2) TNM staging, 3) biomarker status (ER/PR/HER2), and 4) the starting dates of the breast cancer treatment/interventions for one treatment course (Appendix B1).

The data collection tool for Segment 2 was a data collection form. The data collection form comprised of four parts: A, B, C and D. Respondents were interviewed face-to-face using this data collection form (Appendix B2).

In Part A, the information collected were sociodemographic data and socioeconomic data. Sociodemographic data collected were date of birth, ethnicity, place of residence (housing area, village, township or district), household composition (who lived with the respondent at the time of treatment), marital status and education level. Socioeconomic data collected were respondent's occupation and income.

In Part B, the information collected was on the date (approximate) of diagnosis, the treatment they have undergone since they were diagnosed (location and frequency) and the OOP expenditure for treatment and intervention they incurred from the time of diagnosis. The respondent was asked about all breast cancer-related activities they had undergone up until the day of the interview. The activities were: mammogram screening, diagnostic assessments, surgery, chemotherapy, radiotherapy and all other interventions related to breast cancer. For each of these activities, the respondent was asked on the amount that they had spent out-of-pocket. If an activity was recurrent, the frequency and amount spent for each activity was obtained. If the amount spent on a recurrent activity was approximately similar, then the frequency and amount spent were multiplied. This OOP expenditure amount reported by the patient were then analyzed.

In Part C, data collected were on the respondent's estimated household average monthly income and estimated household average monthly food expenditure. The method of payment for the treatment and travel expenditure was also ascertained: whether they were purely out-of-pocket, reimbursed by insurance, has government servant health benefit, received financial aid from organizations or family; or from savings.

In Part D, data collected was on the modes of transportation used to travel to hospital/health facilities, the estimated OOP expenditure incurred for toll charges, parking fees, fares for public transportation (if used), food and accommodation for each visit (if any). Estimated average monthly expenditure on traditional and complementary medicine and health supplement was also asked.

3.4 Combined Data Analysis

The available data collected were combined and analysed to determine service coverage, financial protection coverage and UHC composite index score. In general, all categorical data were analysed descriptively and presented as frequency and percentages. Continuous data were presented as range, mean and standard deviation, as well as median and interquartile range. Data which were not normally distributed were analysed using non-parametric tests. Bivariate and multivariate analysis was done using Chi-square test and logistic regression. All tests were two sided and a nominal significance level of 0.05 was used.

To determine the availability building blocks of the health system, descriptive data analysis was carried out. To calculate the effective service coverage score, data collected using the data collection form was imputed into an Excel worksheet. Based on the hormone receptor status, the type of surgery done and the HER status, the duration between the date of diagnosis and the dates of treatment/intervention was determined. The percentage of respondents whose care adhered to the indicators, the 95% confidence interval and mean duration (± standard deviation, SD) were then determined.

As for the calculation of financial protection coverage, Data analysis was done to determine the: 1) sociodemographic characteristics of the respondents, 2) the average monthly household income, 3) the average monthly household food expenditure, 4) the average monthly household capacity to pay, 5) the average monthly out-of-pocket treatment expenditure of breast cancer, 6) the average monthly out-of-pocket travelling expenditure for breast cancer treatment, 7) the prevalence of catastrophic health expenditure,

8) the prevalence of impoverishment (poverty headcount), and 9) the impoverishment overshoot (poverty gap).

To estimate the average monthly household capacity to pay, the average monthly household food expenditure was subtracted from the average monthly household income (WHO 2010b).

To estimate the out-of-pocket treatment expenditure of breast cancer, the estimated expenditure for allopathic as well as traditional and complementary medicines was summed. This total estimated treatment expenditure was taken as net of any reimbursements (example insurance), financial aids (example civil servant medical benefits, contribution from family members or organizations) and discounts for elderly patients (50% discount for those aged 55 years and above at government hospitals).

For standardization purposes, the estimated travelling expenditure for respondents who claimed to have used their personal cars for travelling, the distance travelled would be determined from the area of their residence and the health facility they attended. Then the distance between these two points was estimated by imputing the data into a mapping application. The application determined the choices of actual routes including the estimated distances. The route with the shortest distance shown by the mapping application was chosen. This travel distance was then multiplied by the number of visits to the facilities and further multiplied by two to account for return trips. For standardization purposes, the expenditure per kilometer travelled was set at RM 0.70 which was the rate for government staff travel allowance using privately-owned cars (Accountant General's Department of Malaysia). This method of calculation was also used in another similar study (Lauzier et al. 2013). Toll rates were determined from the online databases for each of the routes taken by the respondents which had tolls. Parking costs were estimated by multiplying the average value of 2015 the Klang Valley hospital parking rates (RM 2.00 per hour) by the number of visits to these facilities. The number of hours for parking was estimated as three hours at the hospital outpatient clinics based on findings from local studies on patient's waiting time (Ahmad et al. 2017; Ir et al. 2011) and six hours for chemotherapy based on observations during this current study. However, for respondents who had travelled by public transportation, the fares they paid for the trips were used in the travelling expenditure estimation. Food expenditure was estimated by asking the respondent the average expenditure on food every time they visited the health facilities. This amount was then multiplied by the number of visits. Expenditure on accommodation outside hospital during their treatment phase (if present) was based on the rate being as reported by the respondent or as stated in the websites of the lodging facilities. In this study, if the respondents stayed/lodged at family members' or friends' homes, then this lodging expenditure was considered as zero. The expenditure of zero was used because culturally in this country, an individual who lodges in a friend's or relatives' houses does not usually incur any lodging expenditure: the lodger does not pay the host. Because this study takes into account only OOP expenditure which referred to the actual amount of cash transactions, and not the cost (opportunity cost) of lodging, therefore the lodging expenditure at friend's or relatives' houses was considered zero.

To determine the estimated average monthly OOP expenditure for treatment and intervention, as well as travel, the estimated total expenditure for treatment was divided by the duration (months) of treatment experienced by the respondent at the time of the interview.

To determine if a household had experienced catastrophic health expenditure, firstly the estimated net average monthly OOP treatment expenditure was added to the estimated average monthly OOP travel expenditure to get the total breast cancer OOP expenditure. Then this value was divided with the household's average monthly capacity to pay. If this value was more than 40% of capacity to pay, then the household was said to have experienced catastrophic health expenditure (WHO 2010-handbook). The number of households which experienced CHE was then determined.

To determine if a household was impoverished, firstly the poverty line was determined. In this study the Poverty Line Income of RM (Ringgit Malaysia) 930 was used. This was the threshold for poverty for Peninsula Malaysia for the year 2014). A household having income below this threshold was poor. A household experiencing income below this threshold after spending for total breast cancer OOP expenditure was considered impoverished due to OOP health expenditure.

Secondly, basic indices were used to capture the impoverishment effects of OOP health expenditure: 1) poverty head count index, 2) poverty gap and 3) poverty impact of the OOP health expenditure.

The poverty head count index is the proportion that is counted as poor. In the formula below, where Ph is poverty headcount, q is the number of households with income below the poverty line index (PLI), while N is the sample size.

$$Ph = q/N$$

For poverty gap, the proportion of the number of households (of those whose income was less than the poverty line index (PLI)) from the sample size before making OOP expenditure for breast cancer was determined.

$$= 1/n \sum_{h=1}^{n} \text{Ppre h}$$

Pre-payment poverty gap

Where P = 1 if Household income < poverty line, and P = 0 if otherwise.

Similarly, the proportion of the number of households (of those whose income was less than the poverty line index (PLI)) from the sample size after making OOP expenditure for breast cancer was determined.

Post-payment poverty gap $= 1/n \sum_{h=1}^{n} \text{Ppost h}$

Where P = 1 if Household income − OOP expenditure for breast cancer < poverty line, and P = 0 if otherwise.

Thirdly, poverty impact of the OOP expenditure on poverty gap was then determined by subtracting average pre-payment poverty gap from average post-payment poverty gap (Wagstaff & Doorslaer 2003).

Poverty impact = (Post-payment poverty gap) − Pre-payment poverty gap

Finally, the composite index combines the scores from the financial protection coverage indicators and the service coverage indicators to result in a final score. This final score represents the level of UHC. In this study, the approach used to calculate composite index was the one proposed by Wagstaff et al. (2016) from the WBG.

Steps in the calculation of UHC index were as follows. For financial protection coverage, firstly, complements of the financial protection indicators were taken. So instead of "percentage of those experiencing CHE and impoverishment", the indicators became "percentage of those who were protected against CHE and impoverishment". Next, these indicators were rescaled so that they ranged from 0 to 100 with 100 being fully protected from financial hardship due to health care spending. The CHE indicator score was also incorporated with the achievement index, as detailed in the subsequent paragraph.

The differences across income groups in terms of capacity to pay and their OOP expenditure in getting treatment needed to be addressed. To do this, an inequality-adjusted service coverage score was determined for each indicator. Inequality-adjusted service coverage score is the service coverage score incorporated with the achievement index. Achievement index is equal to the population mean multiplied by the complement of the concentration index (Kakwani et al. 1997).

In this current study, the inequality-adjusted service coverage score was equal to the indicator score multiplied by the complement of the concentration index. The concentration index used was the co-efficient value from the concentration curve for the cumulative household income and cumulative household OOP expenditure. To generate the concentration curve, the mean monthly household income, as well as the mean monthly household OOP expenditure for breast cancer of each income quintile, was calculated. From this concentration curve, the concentration index was calculated as the ratio of the area that lies between the line of equality and the concentration curve, over the total area under the line of equality.

The second step was to assign weight to each domain. There were three domains in this study: prevention service coverage, treatment service coverage and financial protection coverage. The total weight each domain was 1. As each domain comprised of one or more indicators, this weight value of 1 was distributed amongst the indicators, either equally or unequally. In this study, for the prevention coverage domain, the weight of 1 was assigned to the domain's sole indicator. Within the treatment domain, 0.5 weight was assigned to inpatient admissions, and the remaining 0.5 weight was equally shared across the other five (outpatient) treatment indicators (hence 0.1 weight each). The equal distribution across the treatment indicators was in line with the equal spending split between inpatient and outpatient care in the OECD countries. As with the service coverage domain, the financial protection domain's indicators (CHE and impoverishment) were also equally weighted (0.5 each) (Wagstaff et al. 2016).

The third step was to combine the inequality-adjusted service coverage scores within each of the prevention domain and treatment domain. For the prevention domain, to combine the inequality-adjusted scores into a single summary score, the geometric mean of each prevention indicator was calculated as follows:

$$SC_p = SCp_1^{a1} SCp_2^{a2} SCp_3^{a3} \ldots SCp_n^{an}$$

where:

SCp = service coverage for prevention domain
pn = the inequality-adjusted prevention service coverage scores
α = the weights attached to the scores.

Similarly, to combine the inequality-adjusted scores for treatment into a single summary score, the geometric mean of each treatment indicator was calculated as follows:

$$SC_t = SC_{t1}^{\alpha 1} SC_{t2}^{\alpha 2} SC_{t3}^{\alpha 3} \ldots SC_{tn}^{\alpha n}$$

where:
SCt = service coverage for treatment domain,
tn = the inequality-adjusted treatment service coverage scores
α = the weights attached to the scores.

The fourth step was to assign weights to the UHC dimensions. There are two dimensions: service coverage and financial protection coverage. For service coverage the total weight (100%) was 1. Of this, 25% (0.25) was assigned to the prevention coverage, while 75% (0.75) was assigned to the treatment coverage. This weight was denoted by the symbol phi (π) (Wagstaff et al. 2016). For financial protection coverage, the total weight (100%) was 1. Of this, 50% (0.5) was assigned to protection against CHE and 50% (0.5) was assigned to protection against impoverishment. This weight was represented by the symbol gamma (γ).

The fifth step was to aggregate the service coverage for prevention (SCp) and service coverage for treatment (SCt) as a geometric mean:

$$SC = (SC_p^{\pi}) \times (SC_t^{1-\pi})$$

This is followed by aggregating the financial protection coverage against CHE (FPCHE) and impoverishment (FPIMPOV):

$$FP = (FP_{CHE}^{\gamma}) \times (FP_{IMPOV}^{1-\gamma})$$

The last step was to assign 0.5 weight to SC and FP respectively (Wagstaff et al. 2016), followed by aggregating the resulting two values by way of geometric mean to generate the final score of the composite index, or the UHC index score, as such: UHC = SC0.5* FP0.5. The final score of the composite index (UHC index score) in this current study was reflective of the level of UHC for breast cancer management in Malaysia. The prevalence in the form of percentages for catastrophic health expenditure, impoverishment and all the service coverage indicators were imputed into the following table adopted from Wagstaff, Cotlear, Eozenou and Buisman (2015) and calculated accordingly. The steps in the calculation of the UHC index score are summarized in Table 3.13.

Table 3.14 Summary of UHC index score

Dimension	Domain	Indicator	As % of domain	As % of dimension	As % of UHC
Service coverage	Prevention	P1	α(P1)	π (P1)	0.5*(a)
	Treatment	T1	0.5(T1)	(1-π) (ΣT1T6)	
		T2	ß(T2)		
		T3	ß(T3)		
		T4	ß(T4)		
		T5	ß(T5)		
		T6	ß(T6)		
Financial protection	CHE	FPCHE	α (FP1)	1-ɣ (FP1)	0.5*(b)
	Impoverishment	FPIMPOV	α (FP2)	ɣ (FP2)	

where:
P1 = prevention = mammogram screening
T1 = treatment 1 = surgery
T2 = treatment 2 = chemotherapy
T3 = treatment 3 = radiotherapy
T4 = treatment 4 = hormonal therapy

T5 = treatment 5 = targeted therapy
FP 1 = financial protection = % protected from CHE
FP 2 = financial protection = % protected from impoverishment
α = weight = 1
ß = weight = 0.1
Π = weight = 0.25
γ = weight = 0.5
(a) = the sum of values for service coverage
(b) = the sum of values for financial protection

3.5 Operational Definition of Terms

3.5.1 Service coverage for prevention

Proportion of the population in need (women more than 40 years old) receiving preventive intervention (mammogram screening).

3.5.2 Service coverage for treatment

Proportion of the population in need (women diagnosed with breast cancer) receiving treatment intervention (surgery, chemotherapy, radiotherapy, palliative care).

3.5.3 Catastrophic health expenditure

In this study, catastrophic health expenditure is defined as using more than 40% of household's capacity to pay.

3.5.4 Impoverishment

Impoverishment is defined as becoming poor after spending on health. A household is considered to have become poor if the household income net of breast cancer expenditure becomes lower than the national poverty line of Malaysia in 2014.

3.5.5 Effective service coverage for breast cancer management

Proportion of women diagnosed with breast cancer receiving preventive and treatment interventions (surgery, chemotherapy, radiotherapy, palliative care) of good quality and in a timely manner.

3.5.6 Financial protection coverage for breast cancer management

Proportion of women diagnosed with breast cancer receiving preventive and treatment interventions; but did not experience catastrophic health expenditure of impoverishment.

3.5.7 Age

Age of the breast cancer patient at the time of the study.

3.5.8 Gender

Gender of the breast cancer patient.

3.5.9 Occupation

Occupation of the breast cancer patient. Occupation means any work carried out by the individual which result in payment for that work. Occupation is divided into three groups: civil servant, private sector worker and not employed. Civil servant is an individual who works in the government sector or has retired from the government sector. Private sector worker is either an individual who works with non-governmental entities or who is self-employed. Not employed refers to an individual who is not working and not earning any income, for example a housewife or a student.

3.5.10 Education level

Education level is defined as the highest level of formal education attained by the respondent. Education level is divided into primary, secondary or tertiary. Primary education refers to completing the level of Standard Six in the formal primary school system of Malaysia; secondary education refers to completing the level Form Five in the formal secondary school system of Malaysia, while tertiary education refers to completing any education level higher than Form Five in the education system of Malaysia.

3.5.11 Marital status

In this study marital status refers to the status of either currently married; or not/no longer married. Married means the respondent has a living spouse during the time of the interview. Not married means that the respondents did not ever marry, or no longer married due to being divorced or widowed during the time of the interview.

3.5.12 Household

A household is defined as the people the respondent was living and make common provision for food and other living essentials

3.5.13 Single family

Single family is defined as the respondent living alone; or if she lived with anyone else, she did not share her income or food expenditure with the other individuals living with her.

3.5.14 Nuclear family

Nuclear family is defined as the respondent living with her spouse, with or without children.

3.5.15 Extended family

Extended family refers to the respondent living with or without her spouse and lives with other family members such as children, in-laws, siblings or parents.

3.5.16 Composite family

Composite family is defined as respondent living with individuals other than her family members but shares income and food expenditure.

3.5.17 Household income

Household income is the estimate of the average sum of monthly earnings of all members of the household.

3.5.18 Household food expenditure

Household food expenditure is the estimate of the average monthly expenditure on purchasing groceries and food items: cooked and uncooked for the household. This include meals eaten outside of home.

3.5.19 Out-of-pocket expenditure (OOPE)

OOPE refers to payment incurred by the respondent for breast cancer-related interventions, comprising of treatment (clinic consultations, surgical procedures, chemotherapy, and radiotherapy) and investigations (radiological or biochemical tests). It also includes any expenses on traditional and complementary medicine; as well as travel expenditure.

3.5.20 Combined OOP expenditure

Estimated combined allopathic treatment, TCM and travel and meals expenditure claimed to have been incurred by breast cancer patients during their cancer treatment period.

3.5.21 Travel expenditure

In this study, expenditure incurred during travelling of the respondent and/or accompanying person(s) from their homes to the screening and treatment facilities is included as out-of-pocket expenditure. Travel expenditure comprises of transport cost, toll and parking fees (if any).

3.5.22 Meal expenditure

Expenditure for meals incurred during travelling of the respondent and/or accompanying person(s) from their homes to the screening and treatment facilities.

3.5.23 Traditional and complementary medicine (TCM)

Traditional and complementary medicine refers to any non-allopathic substances applied or ingested with the intention gaining cure or relief from breast cancer. These non-allopathic-treatment materials include nutritional supplements and meal replacements items (such as specialized powdered milk), special diet, herbs and spiritual-based treatment.

3.5.24 Breast cancer treatment

In this study, "breast cancer treatment" refers to the collective treatment received by the respondent, encompassing allopathic (modern) treatment, and traditional and complementary medicine treatment (if any). Where only modern treatment for breast cancer is meant, the term "allopathic treatment" is used. Where other than modern treatment for breast cancer is meant, the term "traditional and complementary medicine" is used. A combination of these two modalities of treatment is referred to as "breast cancer treatment".

3.5.25 Capacity to pay

Capacity to pay in this study refers to the non-food expenditure, or total household income net of food expenditure.

3.5.26 Poverty line

National poverty line index for Malaysia used in this study was that of 2014, which was RM 930.00 per month.

3.6 Research Ethics

This study was approved by the Medical Research Ethics Committee (NMRR-15-929-25001) and UKM Research and Ethics Committee (Research Code: FF-2012-308). This work was supported by Universiti Kebangsaan Malaysia Medical Center Fundamental Research Grant (FF-2015-308). Informed consent was obtained from the respondents who agreed to participate in this study. All data were analyzed and reported collectively not individually, and the performance of the individual facilities involved in the treatment of the respondents was analyzed collectively and their identities were not disclosed in the findings of the study.

IV RESULTS

4.1 Introduction

Malaysia is an upper middle-income country located in the Asia Pacific region. Population of Malaysia was concentrated in the west coast of the Malaysian Peninsula. The total population is approximately 32 million, consisting of more men than women with an annual population of growth rate of approximately 1.5 percent. Bumiputra ethnicity constituted 68.6 percent of the population, followed by Chinese (23.4%), Indians (7.0%) and others (1.0%). The summary of population for years 2014 until 2017 is as shown in Table 4.1.

Table 4.1 Malaysian population based on year and gender

Population	Year			
	2014	2015	2016	2017
Total population (million)	30.71	31.19	31.63	32.05
Male (million)	15.87	16.11	16.35	16.56
Female (million)	14.84	15.07	15.29	15.49
Average annual population growth rate (%)	1.6	1.5	1.4	1.3

4.2 Proposed UHC Indicators for Breast Cancer Management in Malaysia

The first research question was, "what are the suitable framework, indicators and targets to assess the extent UHC of breast cancer management?" From the framework of UHC monitoring by and available sources, a list of quality performance indicators which were potentially be used as effective service coverage for breast cancer treatment was compiled from various as in Table 4.2. All these indicators were found to adhere to the UHC indicator criteria as detailed earlier.

Table 4.2 Proposed indicators for effective service coverage for breast cancer management

Indicator	Numerator	Denominator	Source of indicator
1. % of women 40 - 74 years old who had undergone mammogram	Women 40 - 74 years old who had undergone mammogram	Women 40 - 74 years old	Malaysian CPG on Breast Cancer Management (2010)
2. % of women under age 70 with Stage I to III Breast cancer who received initial treatment (surgery or neo-adjuvant therapy) within 2 months of diagnosis	Women under age 70 with Stage I to III Breast cancer who received initial treatment within 2 months of diagnosis	Patients under age 70 with Stage I to III Breast cancer	Malaysian CPG on Breast Cancer Management (2010)

3.	% of women under age 70 with Stage I (Tc) to III ER/PR negative breast cancer who received adjuvant multi-agent (combination) chemotherapy within 120 days of date of diagnosis	Women under age 70 with Stage I (Tc) to III ER/PR negative breast cancer who received adjuvant multi-agent (combination) chemotherapy within 120 days of date of diagnosis	Women under age 70 with Stage I (Tc) to III ER/PR negative breast cancer	American Society of Clinical Oncology/ National Comprehensive Cancer Network (ASCO-NCCN) Commission on Cancer (CoC) of the American College of Surgeons
4.	% of women under age 70 with Stage I to III breast cancer who had breast conserving surgery (BCS) for breast cancer received Radiation therapy within one year (365 days) of date of diagnosis	Women under age 70 with Stage I to III breast cancer who had BCS received Radiation therapy within one year of date of diagnosis	Women under age 70 with Stage I to III breast cancer who had breast conserving surgery for breast cancer	Commission on Cancer (CoC) of the American College of Surgeons
5.	% of women under age 70 who had mastectomy for breast cancer with node+ received radiation therapy within 1 year (365 days) of date of diagnosis	Women under age 70 who had mastectomy for breast cancer with node+ received radiation therapy within 1 year (365 days) of date of diagnosis	Women under age 70 who had mastectomy for breast cancer with node+	Commission on Cancer (CoC) of the American College of Surgeons

6.	% of women greater than age 17 with Stage I to III ER or PR positive breast cancer received Tamoxifen or Aromatase Inhibitor within 1 year (365 days) of date of diagnosis	Women greater than age 17 with Stage I to III ER or PR positive breast cancer received Tamoxifen or Aromatase Inhibitor within 1 year (365 days) of date of diagnosis	Women greater than age 17 with Stage I to III ER or PR positive breast cancer	American Society of Clinical Oncology/ National Comprehensive Cancer Network (ASCO-NCCN) Commission on Cancer (CoC) of the American College of Surgeons
7.	% of women with AJCC stage I (T1c) – III and human epidermal growth factor receptor 2 (HER2) positive breast cancer who receive adjuvant chemotherapy, were administered Trastuzumab	Women with AJCC stage I (T1c) – III and human epidermal growth factor receptor 2 (HER2) positive breast cancer who receive adjuvant chemotherapy, were administered Trastuzumab	Women with AJCC stage I (T1c) – III and human epidermal growth factor receptor 2 (HER2) positive breast cancer who receive adjuvant chemotherapy	American Society of Clinical Oncology (ASCO)
8.	Access to palliative care assessed by morphine-equivalent consumption of strong opioid analgesics (excluding methadone) per death from cancer	Amount in metric unit, of strong opioid analgesics (excluding methadone & pethidine) in one year	Deaths from cancer in one year	World Health Organization's Global Monitoring Framework on NCD

All the indicators selected fulfilled 12 out of 14 of the criteria for tracer indicators for measuring the progress of UHC. The criteria not fulfilled were: 1) the target of coverage achievement was set at 100% and 2) able to measure equity. The target of coverage achievement could never be 100% for treatment coverage for NCDs especially cancer. The more acceptable and achievable target would be 80% as discussed earlier. Ability to measure equity is possible using these indicators provided that sociodemographic data of the cancer patients were available.

According to Lim et al. (2014) who adapted the majority of the indicators listed above, the rationale of them adopting the indicators in their local study were that: 1) these indicators were evidence-based, rigorous and scientifically sound performance metrics; 2) these measures recommend a specific treatment modality for a sub-group of cancer patients defined by specific tumor characteristics and further specify a time interval from diagnosis when treatment should be initiated; 3) these measures have been adopted by national bodies tasked with health care quality oversight which has helped standardize the collection of cancer care data and enable the evaluation of the extent to which cancer care in a country adhere with current evidence as described by the performance measures and 4) the measures have helped identify factors contributing to sub-optimal care, so that appropriate strategies and interventions could be implemented to improve the delivery of services.

The financial protection coverage indictors proposed for this study were: 1) CHE occurs when the breast cancer patient's household spends more than 40% of non-food expenditure on breast cancer treatment and 2) impoverishment occurs when the breast cancer patient's household is pushed below the poverty line of RM 930 after having spent on breast cancer treatment.

Save time in Word with new buttons that show up where you need them. To change the way a picture fits in your document, click it and a button for layout options appears next to it. When you work on a table, click where you want to add a row or a column, and then click the plus sign.

Reading is easier, too, in the new Reading view. You can collapse parts of the document and focus on the text you want. If you need to stop reading before you reach the end, Word remembers where you left off - even on another device.

4.3 Availability of the Building Blocks of UHC

The second research question was: "What is the level of availability of building blocks of the Malaysian health system pertaining to breast cancer management?" The corresponding objective was to describe the availability of the building blocks of the Malaysian health system.

4.3.1 Leadership and governance

The role of leadership and governance in cancer management in this country has been held mainly by the Ministry of Health (MOH) Malaysia which formed smart partnerships in the private sector and NGOs (Ministry of Health 2016).

The WHO (2010) proposed 10 indicators to monitor leadership and governance in health. This set of indicators is called the Policy Index. For breast cancer, five of these indicators are relevant to breast cancer management (indicators 1, 2, 3, 9, 10). Malaysia fulfilled all these five indicators for leadership and governance as shown in Table 4.3. There were other initiatives and documents specifically for cancer care including breast cancer which also demonstrated the presence of good leadership and governance of the health system in terms of cancer management including breast cancer. These include: National Cancer Registry and National Cancer Registry Report Guideline for Early Detection of Breast Cancer 2011, Clinical Practice Guideline on the Management of Breast Cancer 2010, Protocol for Systemic Therapy 2016, Clinical

Practice Guideline on the Management of Cancer Pain 2010 and Palliative Care Services Operational Policy 2010 (Azizah et al. 2016; Ministry of Health 2011; Ministry of Health 2010a; Ministry of Health 2016b; Ministry of Health 2010b; Ministry of Health 2010c).

There are also quality improvement initiatives such as the Quality Assurance Program (QAP), the National Indicator Approach (NIA) monitoring program, Key Performance Indicators (KPIs), Medical Audits, ISO 9000, Accreditation, Patient Safety Initiatives and Lean Health Care initiative.

Table 4.3 Availability of policy index

Indicator	Documents
Existence of an up-to-date national health strategy linked to national needs and priorities	• National Cancer Control Blueprint (NCCB) 2008-2015 • National Strategic Plan for Cancer Control Program (NSPCCP) 2016- 2020
Existence and year of last update of a published national medicines policy	• Malaysian National Medicines Policy (MNMP) • Ministry of Health Medicines Formulary of (MOHMF), 2017 • National Essential Medicine List (NEML) • National Traditional and Complementary Medicine Policy • Traditional and Complementary Medicine Act, 2016 • Good Practice Guidelines on Traditional and Complementary Medicine
Existence of policies on medicines procurement that specify the most cost-effective medicines in the right quantities; open, competitive bidding of suppliers of quality products.	• Patient Access Schemes • Patient Assisted Programs

Existence of key health sector documents that are disseminated regularly (such as budget documents, annual performance reviews and health indicators).	• MNHA reports • KPI reports • MOH Annual report
Existence of mechanisms, such as surveys, for obtaining opportune client input on appropriate, timely and effective access to health services	• National Health and Morbidity Survey

4.3.2 Health systems financing

Indicators for health systems financing are a) total expenditure on health, b) general government expenditure on health as a proportion of general government expenditure and c) the ratio of household out-of-pocket payments for health to total expenditure on health.

The public sources of financing in Malaysia are the federal government, state government, local authorities and social security funds. The private sources of financing in Malaysia are private insurance, managed care organizations, household out-of-pocket, non-profit organizations and private corporations.

In Malaysia, the total expenditure on health (TEH) has been increasing annually. The TEH as percentage of the GDP has been also been increasing annually from 2.9% in 1997 to 4.5% in 2015. The proportion of expenditure by the public sector in TEH always exceeded that of the private sector, except in the year 2005 when the proportion of spending was the same (Ministry of Health 2016c).

Total General Government Health Expenditure (GGHE) as percentage of General Government Expenditure (GGE), increased from RM 4.2 billion in 1997 (4.8%) to RM 27.1 billion in 2015 (6.6%) (MOH 2016c). Table 4.4 shows the Total

General Government Health Expenditure (GGHE) as percentage of General Government Expenditure (GGE) from 1997 to 2015(MOH 2016c).

Table 4.4 Total General Government Health Expenditure (GGHE) as percentage of General Government Expenditure (GGE) 1997 -2015

Year	GGHE (RM million)	GGE RM (million)	GGHE % GGE
1997	4318	90131	4.8
1999	5249	10 2320	5.1
2001	7367	130 690	5.5
2003	10 478	166 949	6.3
2005	9709	172 681	5.6
2007	13 686	231 359	5.9
2009	17 471	282 794	6.2
2011	20 091	297 382	6.8
2013	23 212	369 955	6.3
2015	27 078	410 697	6.6

The time series data from the Malaysia National Health Accounts 1997-2014 showed that the household OOP health expenditure was equivalent to about 30-40 percent of total health expenditure. Household OOP health expenditure remains the largest single source of funding (76%) in the private sector for Malaysia (Ministry of Health 2016c).

4.3.3 Health information systems

In Malaysia as of 2016, all the general indicators of the health information systems (HISPIX) were fulfilled as shown in Table 4.5. Based on the National Cancer Management Blueprint 2008-2015, the Ministry of Health has strengthened the National Cancer Registry through effective and comprehensive collaboration with all stakeholders (government and private health care sectors including NGOs), as well as establishing an on-line cancer reporting through MOH's Health Information Centre (*Bahagian*

Kawalan Penyakit Kementerian Kesihatan Malaysia). Also, in 2007 the National Cancer Patient Registry (NCPR) was established. It is a hospital-based patient registry which is responsible for the collection of information regarding patients diagnosed with and cancer presenting to participating centers in Malaysia. It is a tool to provide timely and robust data on the actual setting in oncology practice, safety and cost effectiveness of treatment and most importantly the outcome of these patients.

Table 4.5 HISPIX Malaysia

No.	Indicators	Documents
	Health surveys	
	a. Country has a 10-year costed survey plan that covers all priority health topics and considers other relevant data sources.	• Country Health Plan every 5 years, the latest 2016-2020 • Ministry of Health Malaysia strategic Plan (2011-2015) • National Strategic Plan for Non-Communicable Diseases (2010-2014)
	Health facility reporting	
	a. Country web site for health statistics, with latest report and data available to the general public	• National Health care establishment and workforce statistics (hospitals) (2008-2009, 2010, 2011, 2012-2013) • National Health care establishment and workforce statistics (primary care) (2008-2009, 2010, 2012) • Statistic on medicine (2006, 2007, 2008) • Statistic on medical devices (2007, 2009) • National medical care statistics (2010, 2011) • National medical care statistics primary care (2014)

Health system resource tracking

a. At least one national health accounts exercise completed in the past five years
- MOH Sub-Account (1997-2009)
- OOP Sub-Account (1997-2000)
- MNHA Health Expenditure 1997-2016
- MNHA OOP Health Expenditure 1997-2016

b. National database with public and private sector health facilities and geocoding, available and updated within the past three years
- MOH website for public and private hospitals and health care facilities

c. National database with health workers by district and main cadres updated within the past two years
- Records with the Ministry of Health Malaysia

d. Annual data on availability of tracer medicines and commodities in public and private health facilities
- Records with the Ministry of Health Malaysia

Capacity for analysis, synthesis and validation of health data

a. A designated and functioning institutional mechanism charged with analysis of health statistics, synthesis of data from different sources and validation of data from population-based and facility-based sources
- NIH
- CRC

b. A burden of disease study conducted within the past five years, with a strong national contribution
- NMHS

c. A health systems performance assessment carried out within the past five years, with a strong national contribution
- Implementation of Key Performance Indicators (KPIs) in the Ministry of Health

4.3.4 Access to essential medicine

In Malaysia, there are two medicine lists: the Essential Medicines List and the Medicines Formulary. In Malaysia, the Ministry of Health Medicines Formulary (MOHMF) or *Formulari Ubat Kementerian Kesihatan Malaysia* (FUKKM) serves as a reference for medicines used in public health institutions in Malaysia particularly in the Ministry of Health (MOH). The Malaysian National Essential Medicine List (NEML) is derived from the Medicines Formulary for public sector facilities (MOH 2012).

In this study, the Malaysian NEML (4th edition) was initially compared with the WHO Model List of Essential Medicines (WHO EML) 2013 (Ministry of Health 2016d; WHO 2013d). The findings show that the Malaysian NEML had 22 cancer drugs (including Tamoxifen), while the WHO EML 2013 had 30 cancer drugs. This meant that the Malaysian NEML had 73.3% of the cancer drugs listed in the WHO EML 2013.

However, in 2015 the WHO added 16 more cancer medicines to the WHO EML (Shulman et al. 2016). When this new list was compared with the Malaysian NEML 2014 (which did not change), it resulted that only 47.8% (22 out of 46) of medicines the WHO EML 2015 were available in Malaysia.

4.3.5 Health workforce

The health workforce was defined by The World Health Report 2006 as "all people engaged in actions whose primary intent is to enhance health" (Chen et al. 2006). The recommended WHO indicators for health workforce were a) number of health workers per 10 000 population, b) distribution of health workers – by occupation/ specialization, region, place of work and sex and c) annual number of graduates of health professions educational institutions per 100 000 population – by level and field of education.

Based on the document entitled Malaysia Human Resource Country Profiles 2015, for clinical specialists (including trainee specialists in accordance with the definitions used in the OECD data), Malaysia had only 3.42 specialists working in hospital settings per 10,000 population compared to an average of 14.13 in a group of eight selected OECD countries for which comparable data was available (Ministry of Health 2015) as shown in Table 4.6.

Table 4.6 Number of clinical specialists in Malaysia

Specialty group	Malaysia vs. OECD	Number	Number per 10,000 population
Medical	Malaysia	3785	1.27
	OECD average	7026	5.69
Surgical	Malaysia	4203	1.41
	OECD average	14 810	4.91
Paediatricians	Malaysia	712	0.24
	OECD average	1200	0.91
Obstetricians and gynaecologists	Malaysia	1054	0.35
	OECD average	2996	0.98
Psychiatrists	Malaysia	396	0.13
	OECD average	4133	1.31
Combined total	Malaysia	10 150	3.42
	OECD average	44 092	14.13

Fortunately, there are large numbers of new graduates entering the workforce every year as shown in Table 4.7 (WHO 2014) and Table 4.8 (Malaysian Medical Council 2013).

Table 4.7 Percentage of increase in number of medical personnel 2008-2014

Personnel	2008	2014	Percentage of increase
Doctors	9.11	15.79 (2013)	73.3
Pharmacists	2.32	4.08	76.0
Nurses	19.66	30.79	57.0
Medical Assistants	3.19	4.09	28.0

Table 4.8 Percentage of increase in number of specialist doctors per 10,000 population, 2009-2013

Specialist categories	2009	2013	Percentage of increase
Medical	0.810	1.016	25.4
Surgical	0.832	0.996	19.7
General paediatricians	0.546	0.725	32.6
Obstetricians and gynaecologists	0.432	0.616	42.6
Psychiatrists	0.077	0.090	17.0
All clinical specialists	2.09	2.61	25.1
Public health specialists	0.137	0.155	13.1

As for the workforce for cancer management, based on the National Health Establishment and Workforce Statistics, National Specialist Register database and National Health care Establishment & Workforce Statistics 2011, the number of personnel per 10 000 was unsurprisingly lower than the general numbers, as detailed in Table 4.9 and Table 4.10 (Clinical Research Centre Malaysia).

Table 4.9 Ratio of medical professionals in cancer management 2010-2015 per 10,000 population

Professional	n (2010)*	Ratio (2010)	n (2011)*	Ratio (2011)	n (2013)*	Ratio (29.71m)	n (2015)‡	Ratio (30.72m)
General surgeons	543	0.193	555	0.194	604	0.203	518	0.169
Breast & hormonal surgeons	64	0.023	67	0.023	71	0.024	39	0.013
Oncologists	67	0.024	68	0.024	85	0.029	79	0.026
Radiologists	392	0.139	413	0.144	463	0.156	485	0.158
Nuclear medicine specialists	15	0.005	15	0.005	22	0.007	38	0.012
Physicists	83†	0.102	82†	0.102	na	na	na	na
Palliative specialist	na	na	na	na	na	na	9	0.003

n = number of professionals
* = National Health Establishment and Workforce Statistics 2012/2013 (Clinical Research Centre Malaysia)
‡ = National Specialist Registrar
† = National Health care Establishment & Workforce Statistics 2011 (Clinical Research Centre Malaysia)
na = not available

Table 4.10 Allied health professionals in cancer management 2010-2015

Professional	n (2010)*	Ratio (2010)	n (2011)*	Ratio (2011)	n (2013)*	Ratio (29.71m)	n (2015)‡	Ratio (30.72m)
CDR pharmacist	78	0.028	101	0.035	na	na	151	0.049
Total radiographer	na	na	na	na	3258 a	1.097	3613b	1.176
Radiographer with MMG training	na	na	na	na	31a	0.010	52b	0.017
Oncology trained nurses	312	0.111	230	0.08	238c	0.08	262c	0.085

† = National Health care Establishment & Workforce Statistics 2011 (Clinical Research Centre Malaysia)
na = data not not available
a = National Health care Establishment & Workforce Statistics, Hospital 2012-2013 (Clinical Research Centre Malaysia)
b = estimated based on the increment rate between 2012-201
n = number of professionals

The number of Cytotoxic Drug Reconstitution (CDR) pharmacist was estimated in this study using apportionment method. According to Health Facts 2012, the total number of pharmacists in the year 2011 was 8632 (Ministry of Health 2012), while the total number of CDR pharmacists in the year 2011 was 101 (Clinical Research Centre Malaysia). This gave the percentage of CDR pharmacists as 1.2% of total pharmacists. Based on the document, Hala Tuju Pendidikan Farmasi 2011-2015, the projected estimated number of pharmacists (minus attrition rate of 1.7% per year), in the year 2015 was 12 588 (Ministry of Education 2014). Therefore assuming 1.2% of this total was CDR pharmacists, there was an estimated 151 CDR pharmacists in Malaysia.

The number of oncology trained nurses was estimated using supply calculations formula stated below which represents supply (SYEAR) for the required year while YYEAR represents increase rate of supply. From the literature, the attrition rate was 0.2% and increase rate was 5.6% based on 2011 data (WHO 2015).

$$S_{YEAR} = S_{YEAR-1} [1-a]/100 + Y_{YEAR-1}$$

where: a = attrition rate, S YEAR = supply year, Y YEAR = increase rate of supply

Regional distribution of medical workforce was generally higher in the west coast region of Peninsula Malaysia compared to other regions (Clinical Research Center, Malaysia) as shown in the following Table 4.11.

The number of hospital-based clinical specialists also showed increasing trend in the public and private sectors. The number of hospital-based specialists in the public sector in 2010 was 3768 (56.3% from the total number of specialists), increased in 2013 to 4427 (56.5% from the total number of specialists). In the private sector, the number of hospital-based specialists in 2010 was 2928 (43.7% from the total number of specialists), increased to 3412 (43.5% from the total number of specialists) in 2013 (Clinical Research Centre Malaysia). Females dominated most categories except clinical specialists as shown in Table 4.12 (WHO 2013; Ministry of Health 2014; Clinical Research Center Malaysia).

Table 4.11 Regional distribution of medical workforce per 10,000 population 2010-14

Medical workforce	Peninsular Malaysia (west coast region)		Peninsular Malaysia (east coast region)		Sarawak		Sabah	
	2010	2014	2010	2014	2010	2014	2010	2014
Doctors (total)	9.8	17.91	6.7	11.98	3.4	7.38	4.0	10.45
Surgeons	0.38	0.42	0.22	0.21	0.19	0.21	0.1	0.13
Physicians	0.56	0.64	0.28	0.26	0.27	0.29	0.18	0.17
Paediatricians	0.28	0.3	0.15	0.17	0.14	0.16	0.07	0.09
O&G specialists	0.33	0.37	0.15	0.19	0.17	0.20	0.12	0.11
Family medicine specialists	0.33	NA	0.27	NA	0.05	NA	0.04	NA
Pharmacists	3.1	4.7	2.0	2.87	2.2	3.7	1.7	2.53
Medical Assistants	3.4	3.8	4.3	5.1	3.1	4.1	5.3	6.3
Nurses	15.3	32.2	12.8	25.3	10.0	24.5	8.5	20.4
Medical lab technologist	1.03	1.93	0.98	2.36	0.18	3.13	0.66	2.16
Radiographers	0.26	0.89	0.15	0.93	0.06	0.07	0.06	0.80

Table 4.12 Distribution of workforce according to sex (2011, 2013-14)

Medical workforce	2011(%)		2013-2014(%)	
	Male	Female	Male	Female
Doctors	54.3	45.7	38.8	61.2
Nurses	1.8	98.2	3	97
Pharmacists	30.2	69.8	22	78
Medical officer	42.4	57.6	51.9	49.1
Specialists	63.6	36.4	61.6	38.4

Table 4.13 Number of clinical specialists in MOH who gained postgraduate qualifications in five major disciplines (2009 -2013)

Specialty	Qualification	2009	2010	2011	2012	2013
Internal medicine	MRCP	30	55	67	76	44
	MMED	34	27	31	25	24
Paediatric	MRCPCH	10	13	25	27	23
	MMED	12	14	15	21	26
O&G	MRCOG	3	3	5	5	5
	MMED	15	26	23	19	27
Oncology	FRCR	1	-	1	1	2
	MMED	1	4	3	4	1
Surgery	FRCS	-	-	-	-	-
	MMED	23	17	21	39	33
Anaesthesia	FANZCA	-	-	-	-	-
	MMED	37	47	40	43	46
Total		166	206	231	260	243

As of the year 2014, the number of medical graduates per year has been increasing especially from the private and overseas medical institutions (WHO 2015). Similarly, for specialist training, in most subspecialties, the number of graduates had also increased between the years 2009 and 2013, except for the oncology specialty which the number of graduates remained low (WHO 2014b) as shown in Table 4.13.

4.3.6 Service delivery

a. Service-specific availability

Service availability refers to whether a service is offered in a facility. Service-specific availability is calculated as the proportion of facilities offering specific services. In Malaysia, mammogram screening is an opportunistic screening program. Malaysian women have been encouraged to perform breast self-examination and they may opt to undergo mammogram screening at public or private health care facilities. In 2012, the MOH Malaysia implemented nationwide mammogram screening program for high-risk women through primary health care facilities. Women who have factors that increase their risk of suffering from breast cancer and who attended the government health clinic were identified. The health clinic served as the entry point for high risk women before being referred for a mammogram examination at government hospitals (34 hospitals with facilities for mammogram). Mammogram Subsidy Program by The National Population and Family Development Board (NPFDB), private hospitals or non-governmental organisations were other options for the client. Similarly, if a woman chooses to undergo mammogram at the private facility directly, she could either apply through the National Population and Family Development Board (NPFDB) for the Mammogram Subsidy Program. If she is eligible for the subsidy program, she could undergo the mammogram screening for free or with minimal fee. Conversely if she is not eligible, she would have to pay for the mammogram screening procedure out-of-pocket.

Mammogram is performed not only in hospitals but also diagnostic centres and ambulatory care centres. In this study, these premises (hospitals, diagnostic centres, ambulatory centres) were collectively referred to as facilities. There were 327 hospitals (144 public hospitals and 183 private hospitals) in the year 2015, and out of these, 178 facilities (42 public and 136 private) provided mammogram. Therefore service-specific availability for mammogram in Malaysia as of 2015 was estimated to be 54%.

Service-specific availability for oncology services based on the publicly available data in Malaysia as of 2015 was estimated to be 22%. This meant that about one in five of all existing hospitals in the country offered oncology services. Of these, all of them were estimated to have offered surgical services, 70% offered chemotherapy and 41% offered radiotherapy. This finding was based on the following data and assumptions.

There was a total of 327 hospitals (144 public hospitals and 183 private hospitals) in the year 2015 (Ministry of Health Malaysia

2016e). Public hospitals comprised of all MOH hospitals (including one cancer institute and excluding special one rehabilitation hospital, one woman & children hospital, one leprosy hospital, and one respiratory hospital) and nine government but non-MOH hospitals. Private hospitals referred to licensed private hospitals for the year 2015 (Ministry of Health Malaysia 2016e).

Service-specific availability for general radiology (x-ray and ultrasound) services based on the publicly available data in Malaysia as of 2015 was estimated to be 100% in all hospitals; while service-specific availability for Computed Tomography (CT) services was estimated to be 35% (available in 50 of 135 MOH hospitals) and service-specific availability for Magnetic Resonance Imaging (MRI) services was estimated to be 21% (available in 29 of 135 MOH hospitals).

Service-specific availability for pathology services were available at 14 state hospitals, 26 major specialist hospitals, 27 minor specialist hospitals, 11 special hospitals/ institutions (58% of 135 MOH hospitals) in addition to 855 health laboratories and 5 public health laboratories, while histopathology services and immunohistochemistry test were available in 14 state hospitals and 8 major specialist hospitals (16% of 135 MOH hospitals) (Clinical Research Center Malaysia).

Service-specific availability for surgical services for different types of cancers were available all state hospitals and some of the larger district hospitals. For breast cancer, surgical services were provided by surgeons in various surgical disciplines in consultation with oncologists. There have been increasing numbers of surgeons trained in Breast & Endocrine Surgery Subspecialty who are also well-trained in breast cancer management. As of 2015, there were dedicated Breast & Endocrine Surgeons in eight major government hospitals: Hospital Kuala Lumpur (HKL) (3 surgeons), Hospital Putrajaya (HPJ) (6 surgeons), Hospital Sultan Ismail, (HIS) (2 surgeons), Hospital Raja Perempuan Zainab II (HRPZ II) (2 surgeons), Hospital Sultanah Nur Zahirah (HSNZ) (1 surgeon), Hospital Pulau Pinang (HPP) (1 surgeon),

Hospital Queen Elizabeth (HQE) (2 surgeons) and Hospital Raja Permaisuri Bainun (HRPB) (2 surgeons) (Ministry of Health 2015b). These hospitals also provide 'One-Stop Centre' where patients with suspicious breast lesions will be seen at the Breast Clinic and can proceed with diagnostic tests and treatment. Two university hospitals also provided these services: University of Malaya Medical Centre (UMMC) and Hospital Canselor Tuanku Muhriz (HCTM). All these specialized centres also function as tertiary referral centres for other parts of the country (Ministry of Health 2016a).

Of the hospitals discussed so far, not all of them had oncology services. Of these hospitals, only 22% was estimated to have oncology services. The definition of oncology service in this study followed the definition in the National Health Establishment and Workforce Survey (Clinical Research Center Malaysia) which was: services provided by permanent/resident and visiting oncologists including those hospitals that delivered basic chemotherapy and included services provided by medical oncologists, clinical oncologists, surgeons, ear, nose, throat (ENT), gynaecologist and respiratory physicians with special interest in oncology. As of 2015, based on the publicly available data, the estimated availability of the services for cancer management is as discussed in the following paragraphs and summarized in Table 4.14 and Table 4.15.

Chemotherapy was available at all state hospitals and some of the larger district hospitals. These services were provided by oncologists where available, or by physicians in consultation with oncologists. Therefore service-specific availability for chemotherapy for different types of cancers was estimated at 70% from the number of hospitals with oncology services.

Service-specific availability for radiotherapy was limited to five centres: Hospital Kuala Lumpur, Hospital Umum Sarawak Kuching, Hospital Sultan Ismail, Johor Bahru, Hospital Kanak-kanak dan Wanita, Likas, Institut Kanser Negara and Hospital Pulau Pinang (where radiotherapy services were outsourced to nearby private hospitals). There were no government radiotherapy centres in the Northern Region (Penang, Kedah, Perlis & North Perak) and the East Coast of Peninsular Malaysia (Kelantan, Terengganu, Pahang) (Ministry of Health 2016a). Therefore service-specific availability for radiotherapy for different types of cancers was estimated at 41% from the number of hospitals with oncology services.

Service-specific availability for palliative care in Malaysia was still limited. Palliative care was offered in Sarawak General Hospital prior to the establishment of Palliative Care Units. In 1995 the first dedicated palliative care unit was established in Queen Elizabeth Hospital, Kota Kinabalu, Sabah (Bahagian Kawalan Penyakit Kementerian Kesihatan Malaysia). Subsequently the Ministry issued a directive that by the year 2000, all MOH Hospitals should develop palliative care units or palliative care teams. As of 2015, there were only six government hospitals (including both MOH and teaching hospitals) and one private medical centre which had specialized palliative care units (Ministry of Health 2016a).

Table 4.14 Service-specific availability for breast cancer management at various levels of service

Service	No. private facilities	No. of public facilities	Total number facilities (a)	Number of facilities offering the service (b)	Proportion of services offering a specific service = [(b)/(a)] x 100%
Mammogram service	136	42	327	178	0.54 = 54%
Oncology services	43	30	327	73	0.22 = 22%
Surgery (general)	43	30	73	73	1.00 = 100%
Chemotherapy	32	19	73	51	0.70 = 70%
Radiotherapy	22	8	73	30	0.41 = 41%

Table 4.15 Public and private facilities with breast cancer related services

State	Facility with mammogram	Government hospitals with dedicated breast surgeons	Facilities with oncology service	Facilities with chemotherapy service	Facilities with radiotherapy service
Perlis	1		0	0	0
Kedah	8		2	2	0
Pulau Pinang	12	HPP	8	8	5
Perak	11		5	4	3
Selangor & Putrajaya	39	HPJ	10	10	8
Kuala Lumpur	23	HKL, HCTM, UMMC	15	10	9
Negeri Sembilan	9		2	2	1
Melaka	4		3	3	2
Johor	17	HSI	10	6	4
Pahang	6		1	0	0
Terengganu	2	HSNZ	1	1	0
Kelantan	3	HRPZ II	1	1	1
Sabah & Labuan	11	HQE	5	2	1
Sarawak	14		6	3	2

b. Service-specific readiness

Service-specific readiness referred to the availability of these indicators: trained staff, guidelines, equipment and medicines. In this current study service-specific readiness focused on the facilities which offered cancer management services.

As described earlier, the Malaysian health system consists of public and private service providers. Both types of providers are bound to existing legal requirements, regulations, standards and guidelines on the infrastructure, equipment, workforce and services before being deemed fit to provide services. For public health facilities, they are under the purview of the Ministry of Health, with comprehensive annual key performance indicators (KPIs) and quality indicators (QIs) to adhere to.

For the private health care sector, there are three major aspects which are being regulated by law: pharmaceuticals, medical devices and health and medical services. Regulation of pharmaceuticals comes under the purview of the Pharmaceutical Services Division of the Ministry of Health (MOH). The related acts and regulations include the Medical Act 1971 and Medicines (Advertisement & Sales) Act 1983. Similarly, the regulation of medical devices is under the MOH, specifically the Medical Device Authority. The Medical Device Act 2012 was fully enforced in 2014. The Act specified requirements for medical device product registration, establishment licensing and conformity assessment body (CAB) registration.

The regulation of private health care facilities and services in the country was intensified after enactment of the Private Health care Facilities and Services Act 1998 (Act 586) in 2006 with the gazettement of the corresponding Private Health care Facilities and Services Regulations. Act 586 and its Regulations have stringent requirements to ensure the quality and safety of private hospital services, including requiring evidence of occupational and professional licensing, and evidence of adherence to other related health care Acts and Regulations. All private health facilities stipulated in the Private Health Facilities and Services Act 1998 must comply with the requirements of this Act and its Regulations before they are awarded with the license to operate. This license is to be renewed every two years.

In this study, due to administrative constraints in attaining detailed data required for the assessment of the service-specific readiness in breast cancer management, assumptions on the service specific readiness had to be made, based on the abovementioned availability of a comprehensive administrative and legal regulation of health care services.

Therefore, the following assumptions were made: all the facilities with mammogram had related guidelines, radiologists and radiographers and all the hospitals with oncology services had the related guidelines, general surgeons and operating theatres.

In terms of chemotherapy services, although not all facilities with oncology services provided chemotherapy services but in the facilities which did, it was assumed that all had oncology trained nurses, cytotoxic drug reconstitution pharmacists and cytotoxic drug reconstitution pharmacies; because based on the current legislation requirements, facilities which offered specialized services must possess the corresponding trained staff members before permission (license) is awarded to the facilities to operate. Similarly, not all facilities with oncology services provided radiotherapy services. However, in facilities which did, it was assumed that all had related guidelines and physicists.

It was also assumed that the remaining facilities which did not have chemotherapy or radiotherapy services, had only oncology consultation services. In these facilities, once the patient has undergone consultation, it was assumed that she would be referred to another medical facility for chemotherapy and/or radiotherapy.

In summary, not all facilities with oncology services provided the whole array of oncology treatment services. But in the facilities which did have these oncology, surgery, chemotherapy and radiotherapy, their service-specific readiness was 100% or they would not be allowed to operate. The summary of specific service readiness for breast cancer management is shown in Table 4.16.

Table 4.16 Specific service readiness for breast cancer management

No. of facilities	Domain	Tracer indicator	No. facilities with the tracer items	Mean domain score	Percentage domain score
MMG n = 178	Trained staff	Radiographer	178/178 = 1	3/3	100 %
		Radiologist	178/178 = 1		
	Guidelines	CPGs, SOPs	178/178 = 1		
	Equipment	Mammogram machine	178/178 = 1	1/1	100 %
Surgery n = 73	Trained staff	General surgeons	73/73	2/2	
	Guidelines	CPGs, SOPs	73/73		
	Equipment	General operating theatre	73/73	1/1	
	Diagnostics	Laboratory	73/73	1/1	100%
Chemotherapy n = 51	Trained staff	Clinical oncologist	51/51	4/4	100 %
	Guidelines	Oncology trained nurses	51/51		
		CDR pharmacist	51/51		
		CPGs, SOPs	51/51		
	Equipment	CDR pharmacy	51/51		
	Diagnostics	Laboratory	51/51	1/1	100 %
	Medicines	Chemo drugs	51/51	1/1	100 %
Radiotherapy n = 30	Trained staff	Physicist	30/30	2/2	100 %
	Guidelines	CPGs, SOPs	30/30		
	Equipment	Radiotherapy machines	30/30	1/1	100 %

4.4 Effective Service Coverage

The third research question was: what is the level of effective service coverage for breast cancer management? The corresponding objective was to calculate the effective service coverage index.

In this study, analysis of this data for effective coverage was divided into three parts: effective service coverage for treatment, effective service coverage for mammogram screening and effective service coverage for palliative care. Data for effective service coverage for treatment was obtained from the review of medical records. Data for effective service coverage for mammogram screening was not readily available in the medical records reviewed, so this data was extracted from the face-to-face interview with the respondents. Lastly as effective service coverage for palliative used the international standard indicator, the required data was extracted from the relevant reports and database.

4.4.1 Mammogram screening

From the review of the medical records of breast cancer patients, it was noted that the information on mammogram screening was not available. Therefore, mammogram screening data was extracted from the one-to-one interview with the breast cancer patients. Of the 329 respondents, only eleven (3.3%) claimed had undergone mammogram screening prior to be diagnosed with breast cancer.

4.4.2 Surgery

Effective service coverage for surgery was based on the proposed indicator for surgery: "patients under age 70 with Stage I to III Breast cancer who received initial treatment (surgery or neo-adjuvant therapy) within 2 months of diagnosis". In this study, the effective service coverage for surgery was 86.45% as detailed in the following paragraphs.

Of the 290 cases reviewed, 236 had surgery as the first intervention, 52 had neo-adjuvant chemotherapy as the first intervention, one patient had no indication for surgery and one patient refused surgery and chemotherapy.

Of the 236 patients, 170 (72%) had mastectomy while 66 (28%) had breast conserving surgery. Most of these patients (n= 204, 86%) had surgery within 60 days of diagnosis. Of those who had undergone neo-adjuvant chemotherapy (n=52), 47 (90%) of them had neo-adjuvant chemotherapy within 60 days of diagnosis.

4.4.3 Chemotherapy

Effective service coverage for chemotherapy was based on the proposed indicator for chemotherapy: "patients under the age 70 with Stage I (Tc) to III ER/PR negative breast cancer within 120 days from diagnosis." In this study, the effective service coverage for chemotherapy was 86.3% as detailed below.

Of the 290 cases, the number of patients under the age 70 with Stage I (Tc) to III ER/PR negative breast cancer was 97. Of these 97 patients, 2 did not receive chemotherapy because it was not indicated. Out of the remaining 95 patients who had chemotherapy, only 82 patients received it within 120 days from diagnosis, while 13 did not.

4.4.4 Radiotherapy

All cases that had undergone breast conserving surgery should have undergone radiotherapy. In this study, the number of patients who had breast conserving surgery was 77. Of these 77 patients, only 69 underwent radiotherapy. Of them, 60 patients (77.3%) received it within 365 days from diagnosis. Of the 8 patients who did not undergo radiotherapy, the cause was unclear for 7 of them and one patient had the radiotherapy cancelled due to discovery of distant metastasis.

All cases that had undergone mastectomy and positive nodes should have undergone radiotherapy. In this study, the number of patients who had mastectomy and positive nodes was 173. Of these 173 patients, only 149 underwent radiotherapy. Out of these 149 patients who underwent radiotherapy, only 140 patients (80.9%)

received it within 365 days from diagnosis. On the other hand, of the 24 patients who did not undergo radiotherapy, the cause was unclear for 16 of them, four patients defaulted, two patients had late healing and two patients refused.

4.4.5 Hormonal therapy

For hormonal therapy, 192 patients were greater than age 17 with Stage I to III ER or PR positive. Of these, 181 patients received hormonal therapy. Out of these 181 patients, only 172 patients (89.6%) received it within 365 days from diagnosis. The remaining 11 patients did not receive endocrine therapy and the cause was unclear.

4.4.6 Targeted therapy

For targeted therapy, there were 107 respondents at stage I-III breast cancer whose HER2 status was positive. Of these, 67 patients (62.6%) received targeted therapy. Among 40 patients who did not receive targeted therapy, two had cardiac probes, five was later found to have distant metastases, four patients could not afford, three patients refused, and cause was unclear for 26 patients.

4.4.7 Palliative care

Unlike the other indicators for effective treatment coverage which were currently unavailable, indicator for palliative care was available. In fact, there are several versions of the indicators to asses coverage of palliative care using the proxy indicator of opioid use.

The first is an indicator for palliative care coverage known as "Indicator 20" in the WHO Global Monitoring Framework in NCDs. This indicator is states "Access to palliative care assessed by morphine-equivalent consumption of strong opioid analgesics (excluding methadone) per death from cancer". This indicator was criticized for its inappropriateness as an indicator of palliative care due to its emphasis on cancer deaths and the difficulty in obtaining data from cancer registry worldwide. As an alternative, the denominator was suggested to be changed to per capita as opposed to per death from cancer. Seya et al (2011) put forth a method of calculating the adequacy consumption measure (ACM) to determine if the level of access to opioid analgesia is adequate for a country based on the country's consumption of morphine equivalent and defined daily dose (DDD). According to Seya et al., morphine equivalent is not only for cancer deaths, AIDS death or fatal injuries. Other conditions require opioid analgesics as well. To accommodate these other conditions, Seya et al. divided the ratio of calculated per capita consumption and calculated per capita need; with 22.84 (a correction factor).

As for Malaysia, a review of available reports showed that the average consumption of Morphine Equivalent (excluding methadone) for the year 2015 in Malaysia was 4.24 mg per person (Pain & Policy Studies Group University of Wisconsin 2015). The population of Malaysia was approximately 31.2 million people in 2015 (Department of Statistics Malaysia). Therefore, the estimated average consumption amount of Morphine Equivalent (excluding methadone) for Malaysia in 2015 was approximately 130 kg.

For the per capita need, the calculation is as follows. Three major conditions used as proxy for need of analgesia are: 80% of terminal cancers, 50% of terminal AIDS and 15 % of fatal injuries. Each of these conditions require 6176mg, 6750mg and 375mg of morphine equivalent, respectively. Based on GLOBOCAN data, the estimated cancer death in Malaysia was 21,700 per year (Ferlay et al. 2012), while the conventional assumption was that 80% of cancer deaths require morphine analgesia (Foley et al. 2006). Therefore, for this study the estimated number of patients in need would be 17,360. As for AIDS, there were 911 AIDS-related deaths in 2014, hence 50% would be 455 deaths (Global AIDS Response Progress Report Malaysia, 2015). There were 14,194 fatal injuries in Malaysia in 2013, hence 15% translated into 2129 cases (Malaysian Burden of Disease and Injury Study

2009-2014). From these data, the calculated need for morphine equivalent analgesia for Malaysia in 2015 was 110.6 kilogram. The ACM for Malaysia, being the ratio of consumption and need, was 130 ÷ 110.6 = 1.175. This value was then divided by the correction factor (22.84) produced a value of 0.05. Therefore, the adequacy consumption measure (ACM) for Malaysia for 2015 was 0.05. Based on the definition by Seya et al., ACM value between ≥ 0.03 and < 0.10 is considered very low.

Although these formulae and calculations give an indication on the estimation of the need and actual use of Morphine equivalent of the country, and is used as a proxy indicator for access to palliative care, the results were difficult to use in the UHC index formulae which requires the data to be in the form of proportions.

The literature was thus searched for available studies on the percentage of cancer patients who needed analgesia and received adequate amount of analgesia. Three local studies were found. The first was a study based on a national data of the DDD for morphine estimated only 1957 patients out of 15,000 (less than 20%) with moderate to severe cancer pain received strong opioid analgesia in 2014 (Lim, 2008). The second study conducted in the Oncology Wards of Penang Hospital, where Approximately 86% of patients with moderate and severe pain were treated with analgesics as per the WHO analgesic ladder (Bhuvan, Yusoff, Alrasheedy, Othman 2013). The third study was among adult cancer patients admitted to a palliative care unit in Sabah, Malaysia. Upon admission, 61.1% [95%CI 0.54:0.69] of 151 patients presented with pain. Upon discharge (n=100), treatment adequacy significantly improved (PMI≥0 100% versus 68% upon admission, $p<0.001$ (Mejin et al. 2019).

Table 4.17 Summary of effective service coverage for breast cancer

Indicator	Number of patients eligible for inclusion for the performance measure	Percent of patients whose care adhere with performance measure
Patients under age 70 with Stage I to III Breast cancer who received surgery within 2 months of diagnosis	236	204/236 = 86.5%
Patients who had undergone neo-adjuvant chemotherapy within 2 months of diagnosis	52	47/52 = 90.4%
Patients under age 70 with Stage I to III Breast cancer who received initial treatment (surgery or neo-adjuvant therapy) within 2 months of diagnosis	288	251/288 = 87.2%
Adjuvant multi-agent (combination) chemotherapy for women under age 70 with Stage I (Tc) to III ER/PR negative breast cancer within 120 days of date of diagnosis	95	82/95 = 86.3%
Radiation therapy for women under age 70 with Stage I to III breast cancer who had breast conserving surgery (BCS) for breast cancer within 1 year (365 days) of date of diagnosis	77	60/77 = 77.9%
Radiation therapy for women under age 70 who had mastectomy for breast cancer with node+ (four or more positive regional lymph nodes) within 1 year (365 days) of date of diagnosis	173	140/173 = 80.9%
Tamoxifen or Aromatase Inhibitor for women greater than age 17 with Stage I to III ER or PR positive breast cancer within 1 year (365 days) of date of diagnosis	192	172/192 = 89.6 %

Trastuzumab therapy for women greater than age 17 with Stage I (Tc) to III HER2 positive breast cancer	107	67/107 = 62.6%
Woman 40 - 74 years old who undergone mammogram	11/329	3.3%
Access to palliative care assessed by morphine-equivalent consumption of strong opioid analgesics (excluding methadone) per death from cancer		86%

4.5 Financial Protection Coverage

The fourth research question was: "what is the level of financial protection coverage for breast cancer management?" The corresponding objective was to calculate the financial protection coverage.

A total of 344 breast cancer patients who were receiving treatment at the study sites were approached. Of these, eight were found not fulfilling the inclusion criteria and seven refused. Among the seven non-respondents, two were of Malay ethnicity, two Chinese and three were Indian. Therefore, the final number of respondents was 329, which was 15% less than the sample size calculated (385), with response rate of 95.6%.

4.5.1 Demography of respondents

The descriptive analysis of the respondents' demography status is as detailed in Table 4.18.

Table 4.18 Demography of respondents

Variable		Frequency	Percentage
Age	Mean (SD)	51.50 (9.81)	24 - 75 years
Ethnicity			
	Malay	205	62.3
	Chinese	71	21.6
	Indian	53	16.1
Education			
	Primary	8	2.4
	Secondary	211	64.2
	Tertiary	110	33.4
Marital status			
	Married	248	75.4
	Widowed	57	17.3
	Single	24	7.3
Household type	Nuclear	252	76.6
	Extended	64	19.5
	Composite	5	1.52
	Single	8	2.43
Location of residence			
	Central	263	79.9
	Other than central	53	16.1
	Central and other than central (lodgers)	13	4.0
Cancer stage			
	Early breast cancer	Stage I & Stage II	101
	Advanced breast cancer	Stage III	126
	Metastatic breast cancer	Stage IV	102

Location of residence of the respondents could be divided into two types: their residences in their hometowns and the places they lodged in during their treatment phase (usually the homes of family members or friends). The majority of the respondents' hometowns were in the central region, followed by the southern region, the northern region, the east coast region and East Malaysia, as summarized in Table 4.19.

Table 4.19 Summary of origin and residence of respondents

Region	State	Frequency	Percentage
North			
	Kedah	2	0.6
	Perak	14	4.5
Central			
	Selangor	179	54.4
	Kuala Lumpur/ Putrajaya	84	25.5
South			
	Melaka	8	2.4
	Negeri Sembilan	23	6.9
	Johor	8	2.4
East			
	Pahang	7	2.1
	Terengganu	2	0.6
	Kelantan	1	0.3
East Malaysia	Sarawak	1	0.3

Consequently, majority of the respondents (approximately 80%) travelled directly from their place of residence to the study sites for treatment. As for the rest of the respondents, they were from regions outside of the central region: therefore, some travelled directly from their homes to the study sites while a small percentage were lodgers. These lodger-patients stayed with friends or relatives during the treatment period, whose houses were located nearer to the study sites.

Among the study sites, majority of the respondents were from *Institut Kanser Negara* (National Cancer Institute) and Hospital

Putrajaya (n= 144, 43.8%), followed by Hospital Kuala Lumpur (n= 119, 36.1%) and HUKM (n= 66, 20.1%).

4.5.2 Economic status of respondents

The results for economic status of the respondents were on estimated monthly income and estimated monthly expenditure. The results for income were on: 1) employment status, 2) financial aid received, and 3) estimated monthly household income. The results for expenditure were on 1) estimated monthly food expenditure, 2) estimated monthly capacity to pay, 3) estimated monthly allopathic treatment expenditure, 4) estimated monthly TCM expenditure, 5) estimated travel and meal expenditures and 6) estimated total combined OOP expenditure.

a. Employment status

From the results of the study, approximately half of the respondents were not employed; while the remaining half of the respondents were employed. Of those who were not employed, they were all housewives.

Among those were employed, about two thirds were civil servants or pensioners while one third was working in the private sector or self-employed. Examples of self-employment were baby-sitting or running small businesses (selling clothing items and food at food stalls). The results of the study showed that approximately 60% of the respondents were not employed (housewives); while the remaining respondents were employed. Among those were employed, 54.7% were civil servants or pensioners, while 45.3% were working in the private sector or self-employed. Examples of self-employment were baby-sitting or running small businesses.

Majority of the respondents (85%) did not have changes in employment status before and after being diagnosed with breast cancer. Of those who had no changes in their employment status, majority of them were housewives, followed by private employees (including self-employed) and government servants (including pensioners). Only 15% of the respondents had changes in their employment status. Among those who did experience changes in their employment status, majority of them were private employees who became housewives, followed government servants who became housewives and a housewife who became self-employed. The distribution of employment status is summarized in Table 4.20.

Table 4.20 Distribution of employment status

Occupation before diagnosed with breast cancer	Occupation after diagnosed with breast cancer	Frequency	Percentage
Government	Government	75	22.8
Private	Private	61	25.5
Housewife	housewife	146	44.4
Government	housewife	3	0.9
Private	housewife	45	13.7
Housewife	private	1	0.3

b. Financial aid

The findings from this study noted that about 80% of the respondents had received some sort of financial aid for the breast cancer treatment, while 20% did not. Of those who received financial aids, these financial aids were either in the formal forms or the informal forms.

Formal financial aids were civil servant health benefits (referred to as guarantee letter (GL) as it is commonly known in the general population), private medical insurance or both. Informal aids included contribution from family members, contribution by entities such as the Welfare Department, non-governmental organizations, alms (also known as "zakat" in the general population) and employers. Informal aids also included personal bank savings or savings in their Employee Provident Fund (EPF) accounts.

Of the respondents, majority of them (n = 206, 62.6%) claimed they had formal financial aid, 60 respondents (18.2%) claimed they had no financial aids, which meant they used their monthly income to pay for expenditures, while 36 respondents (n=19.15%) had neither formal nor informal aids. The distribution of the types and categories of financial aid is summarized in Table 4.21.

Table 4.21 Distribution of the types and categories of financial aid

Types of financial aid	Frequency	Percentage
GL	100	30.4
MI	74	22.5
MI and GL	32	9.7
Contribution	46	13.9
Others	8	2.4
Savings/ EPF	6	1.8
None	63	19.1

c. **Estimated monthly household income**

In this study, the estimated median monthly household income was RM 3300 (IQR 2000, 6000). The frequency and percentage of the monthly income is summarized in Table 4.22.

Table 4.22 Distribution of average monthly household income

Monthly income (RM)	Frequency	Percentage
< 1000	16	4.9
1000 - < 2000	45	13.7
2000 - < 3000	66	20.1
3000 - < 4000	50	15.2
4000 - < 5000	32	9.7
5000 - < 6000	37	11.2
6000 - < 7000	14	4.3
7000 - < 8000	13	4.0
8000 - <9000	15	4.6
9000- <10 000	7	2.1
> 10 000	34	10.3

The estimated monthly income was also divided into quintiles to illustrate the distribution more clearly among the study population. In this study, the first quintile contains the bottom 20 percent of the population on the income scale and the fifth quintile represents the highest 20 percent of the population on the income scale. Majority of the respondents (n = 119, 36.2%) were in the 2nd quintile within the income bracket of RM 2000 to less than RM 4000.

Table 4.23 Distribution of average monthly household income according to quintiles

Income quintile (RM)	Frequency	Percentage
1st Quintile (less than 2000)	61	18.5
2nd Quintile (2000 to < 4000)	119	36.2
3rd Quintile (4000 to < 6000)	65	19.8
4th Quintile (6000 to < 8000)	28	8.5
5th Quintile (8000 and more)	56	17.0

However, in recent years Malaysia no longer uses income quintiles in policy-making processes in the country's Economic Transformation Program. Instead the income groups were categorized into three: top 20 percent of the population with the highest income (T20), middle 40 percent of the population with the middle-ranged income (M40), and bottom-most 40 percent of the population with the lowest income (B40) (National Economic Advisory Council 2010).

For the year 2015, the T20 income group was defined as having a median income of RM 11 610 or a mean income of RM 14 305. The M40 category consisted of those whose salary bracket fell between RM 3860 to RM 8319 per month, while the B40 category refers to whose income bracket was RM 3860 and below (National Economic Advisory Council 2010).

The results of this study showed that most of the respondents were in the bottom 40 percent of income group (B40), followed by the middle-income group (M40) and least was in the top income group as shown in Table 4.24.

Table 4.24 Distribution of monthly household income according to income groups

Income group	Frequency	Percentage
Top 20 (T20)	41	12.5
Middle 40 (M40)	114	34.7
Bottom 40 (B40)	174	52.9

The corresponding estimated mean monthly household income according to the three income groups was as shown in Table 4.25.

Table 4.25 Estimated mean income between the income groups

Income group	Mean (RM)	SD (RM)
Top 20 (T20)	12 707.32	6998.19
Middle 40 (M40)	5501.75	1403.47
Bottom 40 (B40)	2140.23	820.91

d. Estimated monthly food expenditure

In this study, the estimated monthly food expenditure has a normal distribution, and ranged between RM 100.00 and RM 2000.00. The estimated mean monthly food expenditure was RM 658.51 (SD 333.09, range RM 100.00 - RM 2000.00). The distribution of estimated monthly food expenditure and their percentages from monthly household income according to income groups is shown in Table 4.27. Based on the ANOVA test, there was not a significant effect of food expenditure on income group at the $p<.05$ level for the three conditions [$F(2, 326) = 0.342$, $p = 0.711$].

Table 4.26 Estimated monthly food expenditure
according to income groups

Income group	Mean (RM)	SD (RM)
Top 20 (T20)	1052.44	502.49
Middle 40 (M40)	671.93	327.77
Bottom 40 (B40)	441.38	269.47

The richer the household the more estimated monthly expenditure they had for food, but the percentage of this expenditure from the total household income was relatively smaller; compared to poorer households as shown in Table 4.27.

Table 4.27 Estimated percentage of monthly food expenditure from total household income according to income groups

Income group	Percentage
Top 20 (T20)	9.2
Middle 40 (M40)	14.1
Bottom 40 (B40)	26.5

e. **Estimated monthly household capacity to pay**

In this study, the estimated median monthly household capacity-to-pay (CTP) for all respondents was RM 2700 (IQR 1500, 5100). This CTP ranged between RM 100 and RM 39 100. The overall CTP is non-normally distributed with skewness of 4.32 (SE = 0.13). However, CTP distribution according to income groups was normal. The higher the income group, the higher the capacity to pay, as shown in Table 4.28. Based on the ANOVA test, there was significant effect of food expenditure on income group at the $p<.05$ level for the three conditions [$F(2, 326) = 254.55$, $p < 0.001$].

Table 4.28 Estimated monthly capacity to pay according to income groups

Income group	Mean (RM)	SD (RM)
Top 20 (T20)	11 630.49	6869.71
Middle 40 (M40)	4770.18	1398.57
Bottom 40 (B40)	1628.16	720.14

f. Estimated monthly allopathic expenditure

Approximately 26 percent (n = 88), of the respondents had no monthly treatment expenditure, due to them receiving financial aids; while for the remainder of the respondents, the expenditure ranged between RM 5.00 and RM 1598.00. The estimated median treatment monthly expenditure was RM 112.00 (IQR 72.05, 245.90). This expenditure was non-normally distributed with skewness of 3.03 (SE = 0.16). The median estimated monthly allopathic treatment expenditure was 4.15 percent from the capacity to pay.

Based on the income groups, the estimated monthly treatment expenditure was directly related to the income group as shown in Table 4.29. However, these differences were not statistically significant, based on the Kruskal-Wallis test (H statistic was 1.8055 (2, n=241), p = 0. 40545 (at significance level p<0.05).

Table 4.29 Estimated monthly treatment expenditure according to income groups

Income groups	Frequency	Median (RM)	IQR (RM)
Top 20 (T20)	29	101.55	37.69, 303.93
Middle 40 (M40)	82	133.10	70.42, 300. 50
Bottom 40 (B40)	130	108.90	75.32, 177.16

g. Estimated monthly TCM expenditure

Approximately 73 percent (n = 239), of the respondents had no monthly TCM expenditure; while for the remainder of the respondents, the median TCM monthly expenditure was RM 112.00 (IQR 61.00, 250.00). This expenditure was non-normally distributed with skewness of 1.22 (SE = 0.25). This expenditure ranged between RM 8.00 and RM 500.00. The median estimated TCM expenditure was 4.15 percent from capacity to pay.

Based on the income groups, the estimated monthly TCM expenditure was directly related to the income group as shown in Table 4.30. These differences were statistically significant, based on the Kruskal-Wallis test (H statistic was 8.3714 (2, n=90), p = 0. 01521 (at significance level p<0.05).

Table 4.30 Estimated monthly TCM expenditure according to income groups

Income group	Frequency	Median (RM)	IQR
Top 20 (T20)	12	189.86	98.75, 300.00
Middle 40 (M40)	39	193.02	100.00, 253.39
Bottom 40 (B40)	39	123.81	51.25, 150.00

h. Estimated monthly travel and meal expenditure

The estimated median travel and meals monthly expenditure was RM 90.00 (IQR 49.00, 146.00). This expenditure was non-normally distributed with skewness of 3.41 (SE = 0.13). The expenditure ranged between RM 10.00 and RM 1132.00. The median estimated travel and meals monthly expenditure was 3.3 % from capacity to pay.

Based on the income groups, the estimated monthly travel and meal expenditure was highest among the middle-income group as shown in Table 4.31. However, these differences were not statistically significant, based on the Kruskal-Wallis test (H statistic was 3.1656 (2, n= 3290), p = 0. 2054 (at significance level p<0.05).

Table 4.31 Estimated monthly travel and meal expenditure in income groups

Income group	Median (RM)	IQR
Top 20 (T20)	75.97	52.55, 141.88
Middle 40 (M40)	103.18	58.40, 152.16
Bottom 40 (B40)	83.88	44.04, 143.10

i. Estimated monthly combined OOP expenditure

The estimated median monthly combined OOP expenditure was RM 242.12 (IQR 140.00, 408.00) per month. This expenditure was non-normally distributed with skewness of 10.16 (SE = 0.13). The expenditure ranged between RM 10.50 and RM 9106.50. The estimated median monthly combined OOP expenditure was 8.6% from capacity to pay (Table 4.32).

In this study the estimated median monthly combined OOP expenditure was highest in the M40 group, followed by the T20 group and the B40 group. These differences were statistically significant, based on the Kruskal-Wallis test (H statistic was 13.4254 (2, n=329), p = 0.00122 (at significance level p<0.05).

Table 4.32 Median estimated travel and meals monthly expenditure

Income groups	Median (RM)	IQR
Top 20 (T20)	263.41	153.37, 420.42
Middle 40 (M40)	281.69	171.69, 497.64
Bottom 40 (B40)	218.20	111.48, 324.04

4.6 Catastrophic Health Expenditure

In this study, catastrophic health expenditure (CHE) was defined as spending 40% or more of capacity-to-pay on breast cancer treatment, based on the definition by Wagstaff & van Doorslaer (2003). Therefore, the monthly combined OOP expenditure for breast cancer was divided by the household's monthly capacity-to-pay.

In this study among the 329 respondents, 24 experienced CHE, while 306 did not experience CHE. Therefore, the prevalence of CHE was 6.99%. This meant that financial protection coverage for CHE of 93.0%.

The results of this study showed that among the respondents' households which did experience CHE, the range of OOP expenditure from their capacity-to-pay was between 41% and 295%, with a median of 81% (IQR 53, 148). CHE was most prevalent in the B40 households (96% of all CHE cases), low prevalence in M40 households (4% of all CHE cases) and zero prevalence in the T20 households, as shown in Table 4.33.

Table 4.33 Distribution of CHE within household income groups

Income group	(a) Frequency of households in each income group	(b) Prevalence of CHE within income group	(c) Percentage of CHE within income group [(b/a)*100%]	(d) Percentage of CHE overall [(b/24)*100%]
Top 20 (T20)	41	0	0%	0%
Middle 40 (M40)	114	1	0.90%	4.20%
Bottom 40 (B40)	174	23	13.22%	95.80%

The socioeconomic description of the household which did experience CHE is summarized in Table 4.35. Most of the respondents' households which experienced CHE were of non-Malay ethnicity, married, lived in nuclear families, had secondary education, housewives, had no financial aids and suffered from locally advanced breast cancer.

Majority of these respondents were from the central region compared to those who were from places other than the central region. However, this finding needed to be looked at in more detail. Although the number of respondents from the central region was higher than those who were not, the percentage of these central-dwelling respondents were only 5 percent from all central-dwelling respondents (16/263); while respondents from non-centrally dwelling respondents was 13 percent from all non-centrally dwelling respondents (9/66).

Table 4.34 Socioeconomic description of the households which experienced CHE

Variables	Categories	Frequency	Percentage
Age	Mean (SD)	54.92 (7.93)	
Ethnicity			
	Malay	7	29.2
	Non-Malay	17	70.8
Marital status			
	Married	13	54.2
	Not married	11	45.8
Education level			
	Up to secondary	22	91.7
	> secondary	2	9.3
Location			
	Central region	14	58.3
	Other than central	10	41.7
Household type			
	Nuclear	14	58.3
	Not nuclear	10	41.7
Occupation before and after cancer			
	Remained working	5	20.8
	Remained as housewife	11	45.8
	Was in private sector/self-employed, now housewife	8	33.4
Stage of breast cancer			
	Non-metastatic	17	70.8
	Metastatic	7	29.2
Financial aid			
	None	1	4.2
	Had	23	95.8
Estimated monthly household income	Mean (SD)	4850.00 (4,142.25)	
Estimated monthly capacity-to-pay	Mean (SD)	2,925.00 (1,816.00)	

In this study, income-related equality was noted. The richer households spent more OOP for breast cancer while poor household spent less OOP for breast cancer as shown in Figure 4.1. The vertical bar plot in Figure 4.1 shows the estimated monthly income for each income group, while the blue line represents the estimated monthly OOP expenditure for breast cancer. In this graph, the income level coincided with the OOP expenditure.

A concentration curve on the equality of OOP expenditure based on the household income was plotted. Cumulative out-of-pocket expenditure (y axis) of the respondents was plotted against the cumulative income (x axis) of the respondents. The resulting concentration curve was noted to be above the line of equality (Figure 4.2). The concentration index calculated was - 0.02. This meant that the inequality in OOP expenditure for breast cancer was pro-poor, which indicated that the rich population spent more while the poor population spent less in getting breast cancer management.

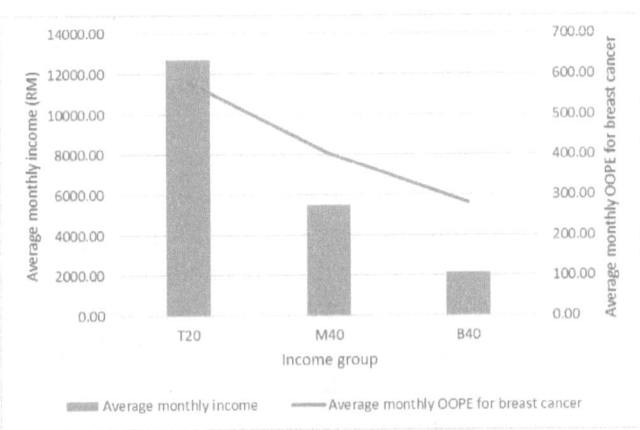

Figure 4.1 Monthly OOPE for breast cancer against monthly income

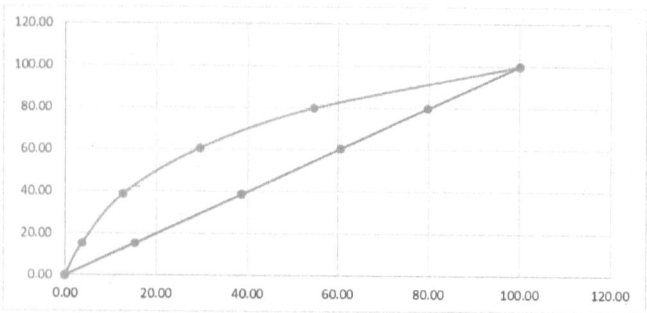

Figure 4.2 Concentration curve of cumulative out-of-pocket expenditure versus cumulative income

— Line of equality
— Concentration curve

In this study, approximately 7 percent of the respondents had to spend more than 40 percent of their CTP to get these treatments, which resulted in them experiencing catastrophic health expenditure. This phenomenon is demonstrated in Figure 4.3 where the poorer households had a larger percentage of OOP expenditure for breast cancer treatment from their capacity-to-pay. The vertical bar plot in Figure 4.3 shows the estimated monthly CTP for each income group. The blue line represents the estimated percentage of monthly OOP expenditure for breast cancer from CTP. In this graph, the higher the household's CTP, the smaller the percentage of OOP from their CTP. This meant that even though the richer households spent more for breast cancer per month, this expenditure was only a small percentage of their CTP. On the other hand, even though the poor households spent less for breast cancer, that expenditure constituted a larger percentage of their CTP, resulting in CHE for these households.

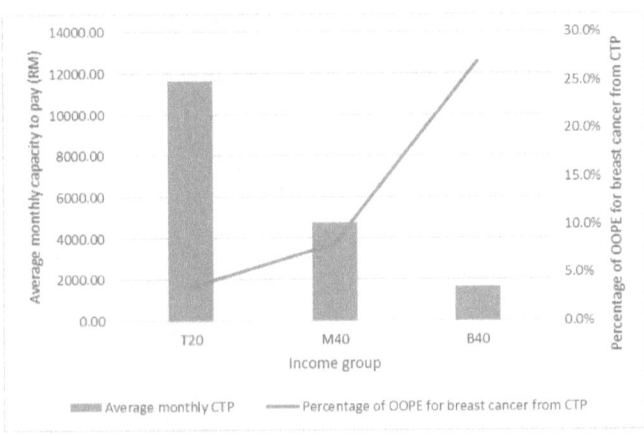

Figure 4.3 Monthly OOPE for breast cancer against monthly CTP

4.7 Impoverishment

In this study, impoverishment was defined as households whose income fell under the poverty line when their OOP for health was deducted from their income. The 2014 national poverty line of RM 930.00 was used, as opposed to the international poverty line.

In this study, 13 households were already poor even before spending on breast cancer management, while an additional 18 households became poor after spending on breast cancer. Therefore, in the total number of households which experienced impoverishment due to breast cancer expenditure in this study was 31 (9%). The mean deficit of income from the poverty line after spending for breast cancer was RM 374.56 (SD 309.86), with a range between RM 19.00 and RM 1169.00. Table 4.35 shows the details of poverty impact from OOP expenditure on breast cancer based on the study by Wagstaff & van Doorslaer (2003).

Table 4.35 Poverty impact from OOP expenditure on breast cancer

Measure	Frequency	Percentage
Poverty Headcount		
Pre-payment headcount	13/329	3.9
Post-payment headcount	31/329	9.1
Poverty impact (headcount)	18	18/13 = 138.5%
Poverty gap		
Pre-payment poverty gap	306.92†	
Post-payment poverty gap	386.43‡	
Poverty impact (gap)	386.43 - 306.92 = 79.51	(79.51/306.92) x 100% = 25.9%

† Mean of (930-hhold income of the already poor) [in RM unit], denominator = 13.
‡ Mean of (930-hhold income of all those now poor) [in RM unit], denominator = 30

The results in Table 4.37 show that OOP expenditure on breast cancer had increased the headcount of poor households from 13 to 31, which was an increase of 138.5%. The relative impact was even greater on the measured poverty gap which was a 25.9% percent increase, calculated from 79.51/306.92. This meant that the number of households below the poverty line had increased 1.3 times more because of health payments, and that health spending adds another quarter to the pre-payment poverty gap.

Descriptive analysis of the 31 respondents and their households which had experienced impoverishment was carried out. The results are as shown in Table 4.37. The mean age of these respondents was 56.97 (SD 9.6) years. Majority of the respondents were of Chinese ethnicity, married, of secondary level of education, lived in the central region, household type was of nuclear family, were housewives before and after the diagnosis of breast cancer, had locally advanced breast cancer, and either had no financial aids or had financial aids comprising of a combination of sources. The median monthly household income was RM 1000 (IQR 600, 1200); while median monthly capacity-to-pay was RM 650 (IQR 250, 800).

Table 4.36 Frequency and percentage of SES status impoverished households

Variables	Categories	Frequency	Percentage
Age	Mean (SD)	56.97 (9.6)	
Ethnicity			
	Malay	11	35.5
	Non-Malay	20	64.5
Marital status			
	Married	20	64.5
	Not married	11	35.5
Education level			
	Up to secondary	27	87.1
	> secondary	4	12.9
Location			
	Central region	20	64.5
	Other than central	11	35.5
Household type			
	Nuclear	21	67.7
	Not nuclear	10	32.3
	Maintained as housewife	16	51.6
	Maintained working in private sector/ self-employed	4	12.9
	Was in private sector/ self-employed, now housewife	9	29.0
	Maintained working in government sector	1	3.2

	Was in government, now housewife	1	3.2
Stage of breast cancer			
	Non-metastatic	24	77.4
	Metastatic	7	22.6
Financial aid			
	None	2	6.5
	Had	29	93.5
Estimated monthly household income	Mean (SD)	RM 1030 (660.26)	
Estimated monthly capacity-to-pay	Median (IQR)	RM 814.53 (IQR 250, 800)	

4.8 Factors associated with catastrophic health expenditure and impoverishment

The fifth research question: "what are the factors associated with catastrophic health expenditure and impoverishment among breast cancer patients?" The following subsections will present the bivariate analysis done to determine association between sociodemographic and socioeconomic factors and 1) catastrophic health expenditure, and 2) impoverishment.

4.8.1 Association between sociodemographic and socioeconomic factors with CHE

Among the respondents, 23 experienced CHE, while 306 did not experience CHE. Chi-square test was used determine the association between sociodemographic and socioeconomic factors with CHE.

As for continuous variables, namely age and capacity to pay, the distributions were regrouped into two groups respectively, based on the mean value for age (51.2, SD 9.815) and the median value for capacity to pay (2700, IQR 1500, 5100).

The factors statistically significantly associated with CHE were ethnicity, education level, marital status, household type, location of residence, income and capacity to pay. There were higher proportions of CHE among the following groups: non-Malays, education up to secondary level, not/never married, lived in non-nuclear households, lived in the non-central region compared to those who lived within the central region, the B40 income group and among those whose capacity to pay was less than RM2700. The summary results of the association between respondents' sociodemographic and socioeconomic factors with CHE are detailed in Table 4.37, where p<0.05 and the reference variables are marked with 1.

Table 4.37 Summary of the association between respondents' sociodemographic and socioeconomic factors with CHE

Variable	Categories	CHE		χ^2 (df)	P value
		Yes (n = 23)	No (n = 306)		
Age					
	≥ 51 years[1]	17 (9.6%)	161 (90.4%)	3.809 (1)	0.05
	< 51 years	6 (4.0%)	145 (96.0%)		
Ethnicity					
	Malays[1]	7 (3.4%)	198 (96.6%)	χ^2 = 10.699 (1)	0.002*
	Non-Malays	17 (13.7%)	107 (86.3%)		
Education					
	≤ secondary[1]	21 (9.5%)	199 (90.5%)	χ^2 = 6.665 (1)	0.010*
	> secondary	2 (1.8%)	107 (98.2%)		
Marital status					
	Married[1]	12 (4.8%)	236 (95.2%)	χ^2 = 7.176 (1)	0.012*
	Not married	11 (13.6%)	70 (86.4%)		
Household type					
	Nuclear[1]	13 (5.2%)	239 (94.8%)	χ^2 = 5.559 (1)	0.037*
	Non-nuclear	10 (13.0 %)	67 (87.0%)		
Location of residence					
	Central[1]	14 (5.3%)	249 (94.7%)	χ^2 = 5.608 (1)	0.028*
	Other	9 (13.6%)	57 (56.4%)		

Cancer stage					
	Non-metas[1]	16 (7.0%)	211 (93.0%)	$\chi2 = 0.004$ (1)	1.000
	Metastatic	7 (6.9%)	95 (93.1%)		
Employment					
	Employed[1]	6 (4.4%)	131 (95.6%)	$\chi2 = 2.462$ (1)	0.130
	Unemployed	17 (8.9%)	175 (91.1%)		
Financial aid					
	Available[1]	22 (8.3%)	244 (91.7%)	$\chi2 = 3.499$ (1)	0.094
	None	1 (1.6%)	62 (98.4%)		
Household income					
	T20[1]	0 (0%)	41 (100%)	$\chi2 = 3.499$ (1)	0.094
	M40	1 (0.9%)	113 (99.1%)		
	B40	22 (12.6%)	152 (87.4%)		
Capacity-to-pay					
	≥RM 2700[1]	1 (0.6%)	163 (99.4%)	$\chi2 = 20.478$ (1)	0.000*
	<RM2700	22 (13.3%)	143 (86.7%)		

4.8.2 Association between sociodemographic and socioeconomic factors with impoverishment

For impoverishment, 31 respondents experienced impoverishment. Chi-square test was used determine the association between sociodemographic and socioeconomic factors with CHE.

The factors statistically significantly associated with impoverishment were age, ethnicity, education, employment, location of residence, income and capacity to pay. There were higher proportions of CHE among the following groups: age 51 years and older, non-Malays, education up to secondary level, unemployed, lived in the non-central region compared to those who lived within the central region, the B40 income group and among those whose capacity to pay was less than RM2700. The summary results of the association between respondents' sociodemographic and socioeconomic factors with impoverishment are detailed in Table 4.38, where p<0.05 and the reference variables are marked with 1.

Table 4.38 Summary of the association between respondents' sociodemographic and socioeconomic factors with impoverishment

Variable	Categories	Impoverishment		χ2 (df)	P value
		Yes (n = 23)	No (n = 306)		
Age					
	≥ 51 years[1]	23 (12.9%)	155 (87.1%)	5.563 (1)	0.022*
	< 51 years	8 (5.3%)	143 (94.7%)		
Ethnicity					
	Malays[1]	11 (5.4%)	194 (94.6%)	χ2 = 10.488 (1)	0.002*
	Non-Malays	20 (16.1%)	104 (83.9%)		
Education					
	≤ secondary[1]	27 (12.3%)	193 (87.7%)	χ2 = 6.321 (1)	0.015*
	> secondary	4 (3.7%)	105 (96.3%)		
Marital status					
	Married[1]	20 (4.8%)	228 (91.9%)	χ2 = 2.177 (1)	0.186
	Not married	11 (13.6%)	70 (86.4%)		
Household type					
	Nuclear[1]	21 (8.3%)	231 (91.7%)	χ2 = 1.497 (1)	0.264
	Non-nuclear	10 (13.0%)	67 (87.0%)		
Location of residence					
	Central[1]	20 (7.6%)	243 (92.4%)	χ2 = 5.077 (1)	0.033*
	Other	11 (16.7%)	55 (83.3%)		
Cancer stage					
	Non-metas[1]	24 (10.6%)	203 (89.4%)	χ2 = 1.135 (1)	0.317
	Metastatic	7 (6.9%)	95 (93.1%)		
Employment					
	Employed[1]	5 (3.6%)	132 (96.4%)	χ2 = 9.167 (1)	0.002*
	Unemployed	26 (13.5%)	166 (86.5%)		
Financial aid					
	Available[1]	29 (10.9%)	237 (89.1%)	χ2 = 3.564 (1)	0.089
	None	2 (3.2%)	61 (96.8%)		
Household income					
	T20[1]	0 (0%)	41 (100%)	χ2 = 26.666 (1)	0.000*
	M40	1 (0.9%)	113 (99.1%)		

	B40	30 (17.2%)	144 (82.8%)		
Capacity-to-pay					
	≥RM 2700[1]	0 (0%)	164 (100%)	χ2 = 20.478 (1)	0.000*
	<RM2700	31 (18.8%)	134 (81.2%)		

4.8.3 Predicting factors for CHE and impoverishment

The sixth research question was: "what are the predicting factors of catastrophic health expenditure and impoverishment among breast cancer patients?" Multivariate analysis was conducted to determine predictor factors of catastrophic health expenditure and impoverishment among breast cancer patients.

a. Predictors of CHE

Multiple Logistic Regression Enter Method was conducted to determine the predicting factors for CHE. Variables which were statistically significant were ethnicity and location. The results are as shown in Table 4.39, where $p<0.05$ and the reference variables are marked with 1.

Table 4.39 Multiple Logistic Regression for CHE

	Variable	Regression coefficient (b)	Wald	p-value	Exp (B)
Ethnicity	Malay[1]	1.294	6.577	0.010*	3.647
	Non-Malay				
Education level	≤ secondary[1]	-0.238	0.072	0.789	0.788
	> secondary				
Marital status	Married[1]	0.759	1.891	0.169	2.123
	Not married				
Type of family	Nuclear[1]	0.295	0.281	0.596	1.343
	Non-nuclear				
Location	Central[1]	1.300	6.520	0.011*	3.668
	Non-central				
Household income	T20[1]		0.209	0.901	

	M40	16.806		0.000	0.998	19599774.246
	B40	0.812		0.209	0.648	2.253
CTP	≥RM 2700[1]	1.935		1.210	0.271	6.925
	<RM2700					

The value of Nagelkerke R^2 was 0.120 which suggested that the model explained roughly 12% of the variation in the outcome. Collinearity statistics showed that Tolerance was 0.998 which was greater than 0.20; while the Variance Inflation Factor (VIF), was 1.002 which was less than 5. These results indicated that there was no evidence of multicollinearity among the variables in this model. The Hosmer-Lemeshow goodness of fit test results showed that chi-square (2) was = 3.109, p = 0.927. As this p-value > 0.05 it confirmed that the model created fitted the data very well. Similarly, in the Classification Table, the overall correctly classified percentage of predicted and observed values was good (93.0%). This value meant that 93% of subjects were correctly classified by the model, meaning there was a good model fit to the data.

Table 4.40 Multiple Logistic Regression Model of predicting factors of CHE

	B	S.E	Wald	df	Sig	Exp(B)	95% CI for Exp (B)	
							Lower	Upper
Ethnicity	1.523	0.477	10.187	1	0.001	4.584	1.800	11.675
Location	1.173	0.468	6.275	1	0.012	3.230	1.291	8.085
Constant	1.025	0.420	5.964	1	0.015	2.788		

In summary, the model shows that a non-Malay breast cancer patient has approximately 5 times more odds of experiencing CHE (B= 1.523, OR= 4.59, 95%CI 1.80, 11.68) compared to a Malay breast cancer patient. A breast cancer patient who stayed in areas other than the central region had 3 times more odds of experiencing CHE (B= 3.23, OR 3.23, 95%1.29, 8.06) compared to those who stayed in central region only. Therefore, the logistic regression equation for CHE is as follows:

$$\text{Odds ratio} = [1/(1-p)]$$
$$= \exp^{(a+BX)}$$
$$= \exp^{(1.025+ [(1.523 \text{ethnicity}) (1.173 \text{location})]}$$

where:
a is the coefficient on the constant term,
B is the coefficient(s) on the independent variable(s), and
X is the independent variable(s).

b. Predictors of impoverishment

Multiple Logistic Regression Enter Method was conducted to determine the predicting factors for impoverishment. Variables which were statistically significant were ethnicity and location. The results are as shown in Table 4.44, where p<0.05 and the reference variables are marked with 1.

Multiple Logistic Regression Enter Method was conducted to determine the predicting factors for impoverishment. In this method, all independent variables were forced into the model simultaneously. The results are as shown in Table 4.41.

Table 4.41 Multiple Logistic Regression for Impoverishment

	Variable	Regression coefficient (b)	Wald	p-value	Exp (B)
Age	≥ 51 years[1]	- 0.580	1.445	0.229	0.560
	< 51 years				
Ethnicity	Malay[1]	1.155	6.856	0.009*	3.175
	Non-Malay				
Education level	≤ secondary[1]	0.769	1.177	0.278	2.158
	> secondary				
Employment	Employed[1]	1.023	2.989	0.084	2.781

Location	Unemployed Central[1]	1.101		5.675	0.017*	3.008
Household income	Non-central T20[1]			0.209	1.000	
	M40	-15.070		0.000	0.996	0.000
	B40	16.957		0.000	0.995	12790288.00
CTP	≥RM 2700[1] <RM2700	16.957		0.000	0.995	23126819.15

These results show that ethnicity and location of respondents' residence were the variable which were statistically significant. The value of Nagelkerke R2 was 0.099 which suggested that the model explained roughly 9% of the variation in the outcome. The Hosmer-Lemeshow goodness of fit test results was statistically significant (p= 0.922). In the Classification Table, the overall correctly classified percentage of predicted and observed values was good (91.2%). This value meant that approximately 91% of subjects were correctly classified by the model, meaning there was a good model fit to the data.

Table 4.42 Multiple Logistic Regression Model of predicting factors of impoverishment

	B	S.E	Wald	df	Sig	Exp(B)	95% CI for Exp (B)	
							Lower	Upper
Ethnicity	1.293	0.401	10.392	1	0.001	3.645	1.660	8.001
Location	1.005	0.417	5.800	1	0.016	2.731	1.206	6.188
Constant	0.874	0.389	5.039	1	0.025	2.396		

The model shows that a non-Malay breast cancer patient has approximately 4 times more odds of experiencing impoverishment (B= 1.293, OR= 3.65, 95%CI 1.66, 8.00) compared to a Malay breast cancer patient. Breast cancer patient who stayed in areas other than the central region have approximately 3 times more odds of experiencing impoverishment (B= 1.005, OR= 2.73, 95%CI 1.21, 6.19) compared to those who stayed in central region only. Therefore, the logistic regression equation for CHE is as follows:

Odds ratio = [1/(1-p)]
$$= \exp^{(a+BX)}$$
$$= \exp^{(0.874+ [(1.293 \text{ethnicity}) (1.005 \text{location})]}$$

where:
a is the coefficient on the constant term,
B is the coefficient(s) on the independent variable(s), and
X is the independent variable(s).

4.9 Composite Index of Universal Health Coverage for Breast Cancer Management

The final research question was: "what is the overall extent of UHC in breast cancer management in this country?" The corresponding research objective was to calculate the composite index of UHC in breast cancer management.

Based on the earlier generated concentration curve, the concentration index calculated was - 0.02. Therefore, the achievement index was = (1/concentration index) = 1/0.02. As detailed earlier in section 3.4.4, the achievement index was incorporated with the coverage scores of all the indicators. The summary for the calculation for UHC composite index is shown in Table 4.45.

Table 4.45 Summary of the calculation for UHC composite index

Dimension	Domain	Indicator	As % of domain	As % of dimension	As % of UHC
Service coverage	Prevention	P1	α(P1)	π (P1)	0.5*(a)
	Treatment	T1	0.5(T1)	(1-π) (ΣT1T6)	
		T2	ß(T2)		
		T3	ß(T3)		
		T4	ß(T4)		
		T5	ß(T5)		
		T6	ß(T6)		
Financial protection	CHE	FPCHE	α (FP1)	1-ɣ (FP1)	0.5*(b)
	Impoverishment	FPIMPOV	α (FP2)	ɣ (FP2)	

Where:
P1 = prevention = mammogram screening = 4
T1 = treatment 1 = surgery = 86
T2 = treatment 2 = chemotherapy = 86
T3 = treatment 3 = radiotherapy = 82
T4 = treatment 4 = hormonal therapy = 90
T5 = treatment 5 = targeted therapy = 62
T6 = treatment 6 = morphine equivalent consumption of strong opioid analgesics (excluding methadone & pethidine) per capita = 86 *
* based on Bhuvan, Yusoff, Alrasheedy & Othman (2013).
Financial Protection (CHE) = 93
Financial Protection (Impoverishment) = 91
α = weight = 1
ß = weight = 0.1
π = weight = 0.25
ɣ = weight = 0.5
(a) = geometric mean of prevention and treatment scores
(b) = geometric mean of CHE and impoverishment protection scores

There are four domains: prevention, treatment, catastrophic expenditure and impoverishment. The calculations were based on the framework for UHC composite index (Figure 2.6). The first step was the calculation of score for service coverage for prevention and treatment as the percentage of their respective domains, as follows:

Service Coverage (Prevention)
= (weight) (score) (achievement index)
= (1) x (4)(1/0.02)
= 200

Service Coverage (Treatment)
= geometric mean of [(weight) x (score) (achievement index)]
= [(0.5)(T1)(1/0.02)] x [(0.1)(T2)(1/0.02)] x [(0.1)(T3)(1/0.02)] x [(0.1)(T4)(1/0.02)] x [(0.1)(T5)(1/0.02)] x [(0.1)(T6)(1/0.02)]
= (2150) x (430) x (410) x (450) x (310) x (430)
= 532

The second step was the calculation of score for financial coverage for CHE and impoverishment as the percentage of their respective domains, as follows:

Financial Protection (CHE)
= (weight) (score for protection from impoverishment)
= (1) (93)
= 93

Financial Protection (Impoverishment)
= (weight) (score for protection from impoverishment)
= 1(91)
= 91

The third step was the calculation of score for service coverage for prevention and treatment; as well as financial coverage for CHE and impoverishment as the percentage of their respective dimensions, as follows:

Service Coverage (Prevention) = π(SCPREVENTION)
= 0.25(200)
= 50

Service Coverage (Treatment) = (1-π)(SCTREATMENT)
= 0.75(532)
= 399.0

Financial Protection (CHE) = (1-γ) (FPCHE)
= 0.5(93)
= 46.5

Financial Protection (Impoverishment) = (γ)(FPIMPOV)
= 0.5(91)
= 45.5

The fourth step was the calculation of score for service coverage for prevention and treatment; as well as financial coverage for CHE and impoverishment as the percentage of UHC, as follows:

Service Coverage (Prevention & Treatment)
= (weight) (geometric mean of SC)
= (weight) (Service Coverage (Prevention) x Service Coverage (Treatment))
= 0.5 [(50) x (399)]
= 0.5 (141.2)
= 70.6

Financial Protection (CHE & Impoverishment)
= (weight)(geometric mean of FP)
= (weight)(Financial Protection (CHE) x Financial Protection (Impoverishment))
= 0.5[(2325) x (45.5)]
= (0.5) (325.25)
= 162.63

The last step was the calculation of UHC composite index which was the geometric mean of the two dimensions' indices, as follows:

UHC Index
= (0.5) (geometric mean Service Coverage) x (geometric mean Financial Protection)
= (0.5) (70.6) x (0.5) (162.63)
= (35.3) x (81.31)
= 54

Among the variables in the abovementioned calculation, the prevention coverage was the lowest at 4%. A sensitivity analysis was carried out to determine the change in the UHC index if the percentage of coverage is increased to 30% and 50%. The coverage of 30% and 50% was based on a study on the percentage of increase in uptake for an opportunistic mammogram program in Belgrade, Serbia over the span of 2009 to 2016 (Jovicevic et al, 2018). Hence, for this current study, using the same UHC index formulae and having all other variables' values fixed, with 30% coverage of mammogram will increase the UHC index to 88, while 50% coverage of mammogram will increase the UHC index to 100.

V DISCUSSION

5.1 Introduction

This chapter discusses the findings of the study, based on the study objectives. In addition, other findings that arose during the study process, which are important are also included. This chapter also discusses the strengths and limitations of the study.

5.2 Framework, Indicators and Targets for the UHC Monitoring for Breast Cancer Management in Malaysia

The first study objective was to develop the framework, indicators and targets for measuring the extent of UHC for breast cancer management in Malaysia. The proposed framework, indicators for service coverage and targets were constructed adopting already available quality indicators on breast cancer management developed by experts in the field on oncology, as well as existing financial protection indicators.

Quality indicators in clinical medicine often originate from CPGs. Adopting CPGs into becoming quality indicators have its advantage and disadvantage *(Walter et al. 2004)*. The advantage is that the results would be comparable between countries because performance indicators are usually based on CPGs which in turn are evidence-based recommendations that often use international standards. However, the disadvantage is that quality indicators do not necessarily account for patient preferences or clinician judgment when scored (Walter et al. 2004). In fact, differences in professional cultures, clinical practice and health care systems between countries could prevent the direct transfer of quality indicators from one country into another country (Bao et al. 2015).

Another study also addressed this issue of directly adopting quality indicators between countries. Marshall et al (2003) evaluated the transferability of primary care quality indicators by comparing indicators for common clinical problems in the UK and the USA. The authors concluded that there were considerable benefits in using work from other settings in developing measures of quality of care. However, indicators cannot simply be transferred directly between countries without an intermediate process to allow for variation in professional culture or clinical practice.

If converting the CPG into performance indicators had to be done, then the indicators need to be applied to a more narrowly defined population than practice guidelines, the target population for a performance measure should include only those for whom good evidence exists that the benefits significantly outweigh the harms and those who do not refuse the intervention. Additionally, any deviance from the acceptable target should be further investigated (Walter et al. 2004). In this current study, the abovementioned conditions described by Walter were fulfilled. The population in this study was a specific population group of adult female breast cancer patients who sought treatment at the hospital, and the of service coverage indicators for the prevention and treatment of breast cancer was made based on accepted international evidence provided by various entities over a long period of time.

Nonetheless in the circumstance where the set of indicators has not yet been determined, the indicator development process should be undertaken. According to National Institute for Health and Care Excellence (NICE) of the United Kingdom, there are nine stages in the development of indicators: 1) indicator definition, 2) indicator methodology, 3) indicator testing or piloting to assess feasibility, impact, acceptability and any unintended consequences, 4) cost-effectiveness analysis (if required), 5) resource impact analysis (if required), 6) equality impact analysis, 7) threshold review for setting different thresholds, 8) indicator assurance to ensure the indicators are suitable for publishing, and 9) consultation with stakeholders and respondents (including patient organizations and professional groups) on potential new indicators, potential unintended consequences, barriers to implementation, and differential impact or inequalities (National Institute for Health and Care Excellence).

5.3 Availability of the Building Blocks of the Health System for UHC

The second research objective was to describe the availability of the building blocks of a strong health system which can enable a country to achieve UHC in breast cancer management.

5.3.1 Leadership and governance

Good governance, clinician engagement, and clear accountabilities for achieving specific outcomes are crucial components for improving the quality of care at both an organizational and health system level.

Countries throughout the Asia-Pacific have adopted pro-UHC policies and strategic plans and many have explicitly expressed their aspiration to progress toward UHC. Some incorporate UHC directly into their national plans, and others have implemented functionally pro-UHC policies (for example, expanding financial coverage or access to services) without explicitly acknowledging UHC as their ultimate aim. In Myanmar, the government has endorsed the National Health Plan 2017–2021, formulating a three-phase plan to achieve UHC by 2030, aiming to increase access, equity, and financial protection (Savedoff 2011) Vietnam has set out a Master Plan for UHC, setting targets to increase coverage levels and reduce out-of-pocket (OOP) expenses by 2020 (World Bank 2017).

Based on the results in this study, Malaysia fulfilled all five of the relevant indicators in cancer management for leadership and governance. Policies, planning, strategies and documents were available. The scope of the Malaysian documents was large and encompassed various levels of care from screening to palliative care. Therefore, it could be concluded that leadership and governance in the management of breast cancer in terms of the Policy Index for Malaysia was good.

5.3.2 Health systems financing

Indicators for health systems financing are 1) total expenditure on health, 2) general government expenditure on health as a proportion of general government expenditure and 3) the ratio of household out-of-pocket payments for health to total expenditure on health.

For the first indicator, Malaysia's total expenditure on health 1997-2015 increased from RM 8.3 billion to RM 52.6 billion (Ministry of Health 2016c). As a percentage of GDP, the total expenditure on health had increased from 3.0% in 1997 to 4.6% in 2015. This finding was comparable to the expenditures of most ASEAN countries during the same time period, which allocated less than 5% of the gross domestic product (GDP) as expenditure on health in 2012, except for Cambodia (5.4%) and Vietnam (6.6%) (Van Minh et al. 2015).

Would the increasing TEH from the percentage of GDP over the years is something that Malaysia should be concerned about especially since the percentage is nearing 5%? The short answer is no. From a review of the literature it was found that the benchmarking of TEH at 5% or less of the GDP was a "recommendation" which has been misquoted many times over the years. This misinformation was discussed at length in a WHO discussion (Savedoff 2005; WHO 2003). The actual percentage which a country should spend on health care depends on many factors such as the socioeconomic status of a country, health needs of the country and the health targets which the country aim to achieve and could be determined using several approaches as detailed by Savedoff (2007).

For the second indicator, general government health expenditure (GGHE) as a proportion of general government expenditure (GGE), Malaysia's total GGHE between the years 1997 and 2015 increased from RM4.2 billion (4.79%) to RM 27.1 billion (6.59%) (MOH 2016c). In 2015, China's GGHE as a proportion of general government expenditure (GGE) was 10.1%, Myanmar was 1.5% and Thailand was 14.2% (WHO Global Health Expenditure Database; Van Minh et al. 2015). As the target for GGHE as a proportion of GGE was set at 15%, this current study found that Malaysia and many other countries did not achieve this target.

Should this failure of achieving this target of 15% a concern for Malaysia? This general government health expenditure (GGHE) as a proportion of general government expenditure (GGE) target was based on the Abuja Commitment when the African Heads of State met in Abuja in 2001 and committed to devote a minimum of 15% of government funds to the health sector in order to address the massive burden of ill-health facing countries in Africa (Govender, McIntyre & Loewenson 2008). While it focused on the African Region, this target also used in other countries to hold governments accountable. However, in 2012 only 14% of governments in low and lower-middle income countries and 29%

of upper-middle income and high-income countries reached this level. So, the target was rarely considered useful or relevant to country policy makers (Jowett et al. 2016). One of the issues was the inappropriateness of the indicator used, which was a proportion of national budgets and not expenditure. If the resources of a country were lacking or if priorities changed mid-year, there may be major discrepancies between what was budgeted and what was spent (Govenda et al. 2008).

Nonetheless, global data suggests that the levels of catastrophic and impoverishing expenditures are low when there is general government spending on health (GGHE) at levels of 5–6% or more of GDP. This was because as the government spending increases, there is less need to consume health services in the private sector, where OOP payments are usually required at the point of service delivery. Therefore, higher government spending could ultimately contribute to achieving UHC by providing financial protection coverage (Xu et al. 2003).

For the third indicator, the percentage of household OOP expenditure for health to total expenditure on health, in Malaysia the percentage was about 30-40% of total health expenditure based on the 1997-2015 time series data (Ministry of Health 2016c). This was slightly above the conventional target of OOP expenditure being 30% or less than TEH in order to achieve UHC and well above the World Health Report target of 15-20% (Xu et al. 2007; WHO 2010b). According to that report, only when direct payments fall to 15–20% of total health expenditures that the incidence of financial catastrophe and impoverishment falls to negligible levels. A 1% increase in the proportion of total health expenditure provided by out-of-pocket payments is associated with an average increase in the proportion of households facing catastrophic payments of 2.2% (Xu et al. 2003). Therefore, the target of public spending of about 6% of GDP should be set if OOP payments are not to exceed 20% of the total amount spent on health care (Mcintyre et al. 2017). In this respect, Malaysia needs to be concerned about the rising OOP expenditure for health in the total expenditure on health which is now about 40%, which is above the newer target 15-20%. Efforts need to be taken to reduce the OOP expenditure on health. Social health insurance should be considered as an option to reduce the OOP expenditure on health.

5.3.3 Health information systems

Integrated health information systems for UHC is expected to capture both aggregated and patient data. It must capture data from private and public health care facilities (WHO 2010, Sahay & Sundararaman 2015). In addition, decision-makers will need information about the state of the population, type of health services provided, contributions to financial health insurance such as social health insurance, human resources, and logistics of commodities, infrastructure and services (Sahay & Sundararaman 2015); so that when analysed, the information will be used to devise, execute and measure health interventions.

Countries throughout the region have set up systems to use intelligence to inform policy. For example, Thailand, Australia, New Zealand, Singapore, Hong Kong SAR (China), the Philippines, China, and Malaysia use health technology assessments (HTAs) to inform policy and decision making (Mohammed, Ashton, North 2016; Sivalal 2009). Health technology assessments have been used to develop the universal health benefit package and the National List of Essential Medicines in Thailand, and the National Health Security Office (NHSO) works with a large group of stakeholders in deliberative processes to foster legitimacy and transparency (World Health Organization. Regional Office for the Western Pacific 2011; Rasanathan, Posayanonda, Birmingham, Tangcharoensathien, 2012).

In Fiji, the health information system (which collects core public health data and clinical-level data via electronic patient records linked to a national health number) provides information that guides decision making in both clinical and management settings The Ministry of Health of Lao People's Democratic

Republic (PDR) began in 2012 to implement a web-based reporting platform to provide timely and accurate data to policy makers and inform decision making, planning, and program implementation. Standardized report forms have been developed, and routine data from health facilities are collected and can be aggregated to district, provincial, and national levels (World Health Organization (WHO) Regional Office for the Western Pacific 2016).

In Malaysia, all the general indicators of the health information system (HISPIX) as set by the WHO were fulfilled. In fact Malaysia has progressed much further by working on to establish electronic health records that would integrate the health records of all Malaysians into one database and accessed by both government and private health care providers, strengthened the cancer registry through effective and comprehensive collaboration with all stakeholders, establishing an on-line cancer reporting through MOH's Health Information Centre as well as establishing the National Cancer Patient Registry (NCPR) to provide timely and robust data on the actual setting in oncology practice, safety and cost effectiveness of treatment and most importantly the outcome of these patients.

As for the geographical information system (GIS) use in cancer management, there was still no known GIS database in the Malaysia. A geo-enabled HIS provides powerful tools to address pressing public health problems and achieve UHC. It contextualizes data from different sources in both space and time using geographic objects (i.e., health facilities) as the common link between data collected by different sources using geography as the unifying element in data analysis. It also helps analyze trends in health data by considering changes in geography through time. Using GIS, an integrated collection of computer software and data can be used to view and manage information about places, analyze spatial relationships, and model spatial processes (Ebener, Roth, Khetrapal 2018).

The way forward for Malaysia would be to focus on the use of digital technologies in the health information system. This is because digital technology has been recognized as being able to improve the accessibility, quality, and affordability of health care services; and the member states of the 71st World Health Assembly (WHA) unanimously adopted a resolution on digital health in May 2018. The resolution urges countries to prioritize the greater utilization of digital technologies as a means of promoting equitable and universal access to health services. The resolution also asks Member States to identify priority areas in which they would benefit from WHO assistance, such as implementation, evaluation and scale up of digital health services and applications, data security, ethical and legal issues. Examples of existing digital health technologies include systems that track disease outbreaks by using "crowdsourcing" or community reporting; and mobile phone text messages for positive behaviour change for prevention and management of diseases like diabetes (WHO 2018).

5.3.4 Access to essential medicine

In 2014 although nearly all countries published an essential medicines list, the availability of selected generic medicines at health facilities was only 38% in the public sector and 64% in the private sector in more than fifty low- and middle-income countries (Cameron et al. 2009). Lack of medicines in the public sector forced patients to purchase medicines privately (Zuma 2013; Zaidi et al. 2013). In 2015, the need for equitable access to cancer treatments in low- and middle-income countries was underscored by the addition of 16 essential cancer medicines to the 19th World Health Organization (WHO) model list of essential medicines (WHO EML). A study showed that of the 38 selected essential cancer medicines included in the 19th WHO EML, a mean of 18.0 (range 2-33) were included in the national lists of countries of the WHO South-East Asia Region and of the 25 essential cancer medicines included in the WHO EML prior to the 19th revision, a mean of 14.6 (range 2-21) were included in national lists; notably fewer of the 13 cancer medicines added in the 2015 revision were included: mean 3.4 (range 0-12). Compared with the WHO EML, there is a lag in the inclusion of essential cancer medicines in national lists of essential medicines in the WHO South-East Asia Region (Chivukula, Tisocki 2018).

In the case of Malaysian, our NEML 2014 had 73.3% of the cancer drugs in the WHO EML 2013, but in 2015 after the WHO added more medicines to their EML, it was noted that only 47.8% the WHO EML 2015 were available in Malaysia in that year based on Malaysian NEML 2014.

Issues relating to cancer drugs in Malaysia as reported in the mass media in the year 2015, were on availability. Claims have been made by clinicians that most of the oncology drugs listed in the Malaysian National Drug Formulary were between 10 and more than 20 years old, not all new targeted therapies were listed, and even if they were, they may not necessarily be funded by the government as it depended on the budget (Boo Su-Lyn 2016).

5.3.5 Health workforce

Globally, the shortage of healthcare workers is projected to reach 12.9 million by 2035. Currently, that figure stands at 7.2 Million. The WHO report (2013) at the Third Global Forum on Human Resource for Health indicated that, if not addressed, the shortages identified in the report will have serious implications on the health of billions of people across the world (WHO 3rd Global Forum

In this current study based on the available data, for the year 2013 the ratios of doctors in the medical specialty group was 0.127 per 1000 population; the surgical specialty group was 0.141 and the combined total was 0.342 per 1000 population. These ratios were lower than the SDG target of 4.45 per 1000 population.

Based on the available and calculated data for the year 2015, in Malaysia the ratios between doctors and the population were unsurprisingly far lower for cancer-related specialties if the threshold for SDG of 4.45 skilled medical personnel per 1000 was used. The ratio of general surgeons to 1000 population was 0.0169, breast and hormonal surgeons (0.0013 per 1000 population), oncologists (0.0026 per 1000 population), radiologists (0.0158 per 1000 population), nuclear medicine specialists (0.0012 per 1000 population), palliative care specialists (0.0003 per 1000 population).

The Health Workforce Requirements for Universal Health Coverage and the Sustainable Development Goals (2016) proposed the annual average exponential growth rate (AEGR) in the size of the health workforce that would be needed to eliminate the needs-based shortages by 2030. For Malaysia, being a high middle-income country, the AEGR should be about 1-5%. On the other hand, by virtue of being in the Western Pacific Region the AEGR should be about 5-15%.

Given the nature of most of patients in Malaysia presenting at Stage 2 and above, a large proportion of patients will require adjuvant chemotherapy and radiotherapy. However, there is a shortage in the availability of oncologists. This is not helped by the fact that those trained by the Ministry of Health have resigned to work in the private sector. To address this brain-drain, the Ministry of Health has continued to expand its training program to produce more oncologists. In addition to the Master of Clinical Oncology which started in 2002, efforts are being taken together between Universities, MOH staff and Professional Society to write a National Curriculum for the training of Clinical Oncologists outside the university. This will further improve the capacity of the country to train oncologists locally Ministry of Health (2015b).

5.3.6 Health service delivery

Health service delivery in Malaysia in terms of breast cancer management needs to be improved. Service-specific availability for mammogram in Malaysia as of 2015 was estimated to be 54%. This meant that about half of existing hospitals in the country offered mammogram services. Service-specific availability for oncology services as of 2015 was estimated to be 22%. This meant that about one in five of all existing hospitals in the country offered oncology services. Of these, all of them were estimated to have offered surgical services, 70% offered chemotherapy and 41% offered radiotherapy. Service-specific availability for radiotherapy for different types of cancers was estimated at 41% from the number of hospitals with oncology services. Service-specific availability for palliative care in Malaysia was still limited.

The WHO has recommended that every country aim to have at least one publicly supported cancer center that advances the broad objectives of control; provides exemplary patient care, appropriate to local circumstances and resources; and concentrates the specialized human and technical resources of the country (Gralow et al. 2012; Atun et al. 2012). Based on this recommendation, Malaysia had achieved this basic aim. However, because most of the current facilities are in large cities of the west coast of the Peninsula Malaysia, the availability of facilities with cancer treatment should be increased and the distribution of these facilities needs to be improved.

5.4 Service Coverage for Breast Cancer Management

The third research question was: what is the level of effective service coverage for breast cancer management? The corresponding objective was to calculate the effective service coverage index. Effective service coverage for breast cancer based on the indicators used in this study is generally good, above 80%, which was the recommended target for service coverage for NCDs.

5.4.1 Mammogram screening

According to the National Health and Morbidity Survey (NHMS) 2006, the national uptake of mammogram screening was 7.6%, while according to an unpublished data from the National Population and Family Development Board (NPFDB and the Ministry of Health Malaysia (2007 - 15), the lowest uptake of mammogram screening was 0.47% in Kelantan, while the highest was 25.8% in Kuala Lumpur among women in the 40-74-year age group.

Currently in Malaysia, mammogram screening is an opportunistic screening effort, purely dependent upon the awareness of the woman about her breast health, motivation level of her to seek medical consultation and the (spatial and non-spatial) accessibility of the mammogram facilities.

Beginning in 2012, the mammogram screening for high-risk women was conducted as a structured program in Ministry of Health facilities, where women who attended the government clinics and have factors of increased risk of breast cancer were identified. These high-risk women would be offered to undergo mammogram examination at government hospitals or through the Mammogram Subsidy Program by the National Population and Family Development Board (NPFDB); or at private hospital or non-governmental organizations.

In 2015, number of new cases of high-risk women registered was 24 199 and 20 457 (84.5%) were referred for mammogram screening. Of the women who were referred for mammogram screening, 20 345 (99.4%) of them had undergone the screening and 94 (0.46%) of the women were confirmed to have cancer (Ministry of Health (2016a).

5.4.2 Initial treatment

In this study, most of the respondents (n = 204, 86.0%) had surgery within two months of diagnosis. The mean time between diagnosis and surgery was 26 days. This finding was comparable to the local nationwide study by Lim et al. (2014), where 89% of patients had surgery with a mean time from diagnosis to surgery of 25 days, and only 25% of patients underwent breast conserving surgery. A similar result was also found in a study in Brazil, that 81% of patients had surgery within 2 months of being diagnosed (Souza et al. 2015). These percentages (in the 80% range) were slightly lower than that of the UK standard whereby in England the target is 85% and Scotland, Wales, Northern Ireland the target is 95% for the receipt of first treatment following referral of 62 days (Cancer Research UK).

5.4.3 Chemotherapy

In this study the adherence to the indicator, adjuvant multi-agent (combination) chemotherapy within 120 days of date of diagnosis was 86%, with mean time of 64 days. Hughes et al. (2009) in their study in the USA, found that treatment for 87% of patients met the quality measure of 120 days of date of diagnosis. The local study by Lim et al. (2014) also showed similar results with the adherence of 75% with the mean time of 61 days. Therefore, the service coverage for chemotherapy for breast cancer in Malaysia based on the findings of this current study was comparable to studies in North America and a more recent local study.

5.4.4 Radiotherapy

In this study the adherence to the indicator, radiation therapy for women who had breast conservation surgery within 1 year (365 days) of date of diagnosis was 84%, with mean time of 234 days. while radiation therapy for women who had mastectomy within 1 year (365 days) of date of diagnosis was 81%, with mean time of 243 days. The more recent study by Lim et al. (2014) also showed almost similar results with the adherence of 77% and 81% respectively. In general, the service coverage for radiotherapy for breast cancer in Malaysia based on the findings of this current study was good and comparable to a more recent local study. Both studies show that the adherence to the indicators was approximately 80%, which could be considered good as the target set by ASCO was 90%.

5.4.5 Hormone therapy

In this study the adherence to the indicator, tamoxifen or aromatase inhibitor for women within 1 year (365 days) of diagnosis was 90%. The more recent study by Lim et al. (2014) also showed almost similar results with the adherence of 76%. The target set by ASCO was 90%. Therefore, the service coverage for hormone therapy for breast cancer in Malaysia based on the findings of this current study was good.

5.4.6 Targeted therapy

In this study the adherence to the indicator, Trastuzumab therapy for with positive breast cancer was 62%. The local study by Lim et al. (2014) showed lower results with the adherence of 19%. According to Lim et al. (2014) for patients with HER2 positive cancer, access to targeted therapy (trastuzumab) was very limited; which was entirely due to the high cost and inadequate public funding for the treatment.

The reason for the difference in findings between the current study and the study by Lim et al. (2014) could be due to the difference in study sites involved. In this current study the study sites were government hospitals only, while in the other study, study sites were two government facilities and six private facilities. In Malaysia trastuzumab was more accessible in government facilities (although still limited) compared to the private facilities. Therefore, there may be higher accessibility due to availability of budgetary allocation for trastuzumab for eligible patients in government facilities. On the contrary, trastuzumab in the private facilities are expensive and could potentially be obtained if the patients have medical insurance scheme which include such types of medications. Although not officially quantified, this current study did detect the migration of patients from the private to government facilities solely for the consideration of eligibility for trastuzumab. This scenario was comparable to a multinational study which showed that common barriers to the use of trastuzumab included issues related to insurance coverage, drug availability and cost to the patient (Lammers et al. 2014).

In terms of the level of coverage, the achievement of coverage for trastuzumab of 62% in this study could not be further commented on as there was no set target for it. The figure however could be used to monitor coverage trend over the years and appropriate measures could then be formulated to address the increase or decrease in trend of coverage. This monitoring is even more necessary now that trastuzumab has been added into the WHO Essential Medicine List in 2016.

5.4.7 Palliative care

There have been lack of quality indicators and absence of routine data collection to show the equity of access and coverage for palliative care and existing indicators for palliation are not sufficiently comparable or reliable measures of coverage (Worldwide Hospice Palliative Care Alliance 2014; WHO 2014a).

The lack of quality indicators for palliative care could be due to the vast scope of palliative care based on its definition. Palliative care not only covers pain relief but psychological, emotional, spiritual and social support as well for the patients and their families, most of which are intangible variables. Moreover, palliative care is given not at the hospital level only but also community and even home level, rendering the collection of objective data, challenging.

It is noted that one common requirement in all circumstances of palliative care is the need for pain relief, such as morphine. For the monitoring of the global non-communicable diseases action plan, it has been proposed that morphine-equivalent consumption of strong opioid analgesics per death from cancer be used as a proxy indicator of access and coverage. Data was to be obtained from administrative data on morphine consumption and estimated numbers of deaths from cancer (World Health Assembly 2013). This indicator was then used as Indicator 20 in the WHO Global Monitoring Framework in NCDs, stated as "Access to palliative care assessed by morphine equivalent consumption of strong opioid analgesics (excluding methadone & pethidine) per capita". It is not mandatory that countries report on this indicator. To date this is only indicator agreed by the UN as part of the global monitoring of hospice and palliative care which was the indicator for the Global Action Plan on Non-Communicable Diseases (WHO 2013b).

It was based on this global recognition of the use of morphine as an indicator to gauge the access to palliative care, that this current study applied the same indicator for the service coverage of palliative care. From the available data for Malaysia, it was noted that the morphine availability in Malaysia has been adequate to cater to all cancer patients in need of opioid analgesia so far.

Nonetheless, palliative care in Malaysia warrants attention from ministerial level right to the community level. This is because apart from accessibility to pain relief, other aspects of palliative care in the country still need improvement. Based on the estimated need for palliative care the-end-of-life for adults in 2012, approximately 55 000 Malaysians needed palliative care, with almost 18 000 of them cancer patients (Hospis Malaysia).

The Quality of Death Index is a more recent index for palliative care service. This index was developed by the Economist Intelligence Unit (EIU) in 2010 and was later commissioned by the Lien Foundation, a Singaporean philanthropic organization. In 2010 data was collected for 24 indicators in four categories in 40 countries. In 2015 data was collected among 80 countries using the newer version of 20 indicators in five categories. The categories are: palliative and healthcare environment, human resources, affordability of care, quality of care and community engagement. Of the 80 countries in 2015, Malaysia ranked at 38. The individual ranking for Malaysia was as follows: basic end-of-life healthcare environment (rank 42/80); human resource (rank 40/80); affordability of end-of-life care (rank 45/80); quality of end-of-life care (rank 45/80) and community engagement (rank 45/80). The country with the best quality of death index was the United Kingdom while Singapore ranked at 12 and Thailand at 44 (Unit 2015).

For palliative care in Malaysia, there were 29 government hospitals with palliative care units in the year 2013, but of these only three had specialist palliative care. Common challenges of palliative care in the country include: 1) lack of dedicated and trained health care personnel in palliative care, 2) limited educational and training resources, 3) lack of awareness of the need and role of palliative care, 4) lack of community palliative care services, 5) limited access to palliative care drugs such as opioid analgesics 6) limited social services and supportive network for cancer patients and 7) insufficient research data on palliative care needs (Ministry of Health 2016a).

5.5 Financial Protection Coverage for Breast Cancer Management

Data for the estimation of financial protection coverage was obtained from respondents. Several issues pertaining to the data collection method are discussed in the following subsections.

5.5.1 Sample size

The sample size of 390 for this study was based on the prevalence of CHE in the ACTION study (2015). However, the actual sample size required for this study could have been lower than calculated. This was because the ACTION study's CHE prevalence was based upon the findings of CHE among the ASEAN countries and not Malaysia specifically. The ASEAN countries involved were Cambodia, Indonesia, Laos, Myanmar, the Philippines, Thailand, Vietnam and Malaysia. These ASEAN countries had various types of health system and had lower socioeconomic status than Malaysia. Therefore, it is possible that the prevalence of CHE from that study (48% for all cancers, 60% for breast cancer) was higher than that of Malaysia's alone. Additionally, the reference threshold for catastrophic health expenditure used in the ACTION study was ≥ 30% of household income, which was not the same as this current study (> 40% of capacity-to-pay).

5.5.2 Response rate

The response rate in this study was of approximately 95%, which was comparable to other studies: recruitment rate of 85% in the study by Lim et al. (2015), recruitment rate of 71% in the ACTION study, and the recruitment rate of 90% in the CEA of HPV vaccination study had (ACTION study 2015; Ezat & Syed Aljunid 2010).

5.5.3 Sampling method

In this study purposive sampling method of homogenous sampling technique was used. This sampling method was chosen because the research questions that were being addressed were specific to the characteristics of the group of interest. To reduce potential researcher bias, inclusion and exclusion criteria lists were used. The limitation of this method, however, is that the results may not be generalized to all breast cancer patients who did not fulfil the inclusion criteria.

5.5.4 Respondent sociodemographic status

a. Age

The results show that mean age was 51.50 (SD 9.81) years. This finding was like the study by Lim et al. (2014) which was 53 years (SD 11), and the ACTION Study Group (2015) which was 52 years.

b. Ethnicity

Ethnically, most of the respondents in this study were Malays followed by Chinese and Indian. This distribution of ethnicity differed from that in the National Cancer Registry Report 2007-2011 which showed that the prevalence of breast cancer was highest among the Chinese, followed by the Indians and the Malays. In this current study the ethnic distribution was as such may be because during the data collection period, more Malay patients were present and more willing to participate compared to other ethnic groups.

c. Education level

The results showed that most of the respondents (64.2%) reported having had highest education level being secondary level education, followed by tertiary level education, and primary level education. This finding was comparable to the ACTION study (2015) results in which 61% of their respondents had attained at least secondary education.

d. Marital status

In terms of marital status of the respondents, approximately 75% of the respondents were living with their spouses; about 20% of respondents were widowed, while approximately 5% of respondents were never married. This finding was comparable to the ACTION study (2015) results in which 77 % of their respondents were married.

e. Household type

In this study, majority of the respondents (76.6%) lived in the nuclear family type where the respondent lived with her spouse with or without their children; whereas the remainder of the respondents lived in other family types. These other family types were 1) extended family where respondent lived with nuclear family members plus other family members or with other family members only (19.5%), 2) composite family where respondents lived with friends (1.5%) or 3) single where the respondent lived alone (2.4%). This finding was slightly higher than the study based on the 2010 Malaysian population census: out of the 6.3 million private households in Malaysia in 2010, 62.3% were nucleus family households and 32.6% were extended family households (Chai & Hamid 2015).

f. Place of residence

Logistically, majority of the respondents lived in the central region, followed by the southern region, the northern region, the east coast region and East Malaysia. Although not formally addressed in this study, the reasons for respondents from outside central/west coast region to attend the study sites for treatment was noted during the interviewing process. The reasons included: there were no hospitals/service available in their hometown and they lived alone but preferred to live their children for company, logistic reasons, social and financial support during the treatment phase.

g. Lodging

In terms of travel, majority of the respondents travelled directly from their places of residence to the study sites for treatment. Almost 80% of these respondents were from the central region.

Among the rest of the respondents, they were from regions outside of the central region: some travelled directly from their homes to the study sites while a small percentage chose to stay with relatives who were located nearer to the study sites during the treatment period. This meant that this group of lodging respondents had travelled from their original place of residences to their relative's house and then travelled from the relative's house to the study sites for treatment.

In this study, the respondents stayed/lodged at family members' or friends' homes, and this lodging expenditure was considered as zero. The expenditure of zero was used because culturally in this country, an individual who lodges in a friend's or relatives' houses does not usually incur any lodging expenditure: the lodger does not pay the host. Because this study takes into account only OOP *expenditure* which referred to the *actual amount of cash transactions,* and not the cost (opportunity cost) of lodging, therefore the lodging expenditure at friend's or relatives' houses was considered as zero.

h. Cancer stage

The results also showed that the percentages of respondents were almost equally distributed among the three categories of breast cancer at the time of the study: early breast cancer, advanced breast cancer and metastatic breast cancer (31%, 38% and 31% respectively).

5.5.5 Respondent socioeconomic status

a. Employment status

In this current study there were no changes in employment status in about 85% of the respondents. Many of them (52%) were housewives, 26% were government servants or pensioners and 22% were private employees or self-employed. Changes in employment status were only experienced among 15% of the respondents, which was from being employed to not being employed (became housewives).

The findings of this current study were like the population-based cohort study which showed that after three years of diagnosis, 21% of breast cancer survivors became unemployed compared to women in the comparison group (15%) not diagnosed with cancer (Maunsell et al. 2004). In another study, 30% were no longer working at the time of the follow-up survey done four years after diagnosis (Jagsi et al. 2014). A cross-sectional study in Japan showed that 29.5% of breast cancer survivors lost their jobs after breast cancer diagnosis (Saito et al 2014). One study reported that 82% of women who had worked before their breast cancer diagnosis returned to work at a median follow-up of 36 months (Fantoni et al. 2010). Studies on employment status also found that chemotherapy was significantly associated with unemployment. It was found that women receiving chemotherapy had 1.4-1.8 times greater risks of experiencing a change in employment versus women not receiving chemotherapy (Hasset et al. 2009; Jagsi et al. 2014).

b. Financial aid

The most common form of financial aid in this study was the government servant medical benefit. This meant that the respondent received free medical treatment because she was civil servant or was related to a civil servant. This finding was not surprising as the study sites were all government hospitals. The next most common form of financial aid was medical insurance. Having financial aid was common in cancer cases. In a study using data from a randomized household survey in Pakistan, 27.1% of those who sought care for cancer at private facilities were found to finance their care through unsecured loans, while 7.1% relied on assistance from others (Mahmood, & Ali 2002). Another study in India found that the main financial coping strategies used by breast cancer patients were saving (74%), borrowing at low rate of interest (88%), social nets (55%), and selling financial assets (30%) (Jain & Mukherjee 2016).

c. **Estimated monthly household income**

The result of the study found that the estimated median monthly household income was RM3300 (IQR 2000, 6000). This value was lower than that reported by the Department of Statistics Malaysia (DOSM) between the years 2012 and 2016. DOSM reported that the median monthly household income was RM 3626 (2012), RM 4585 (2014) and RM 5228 (2016) (Department of Statistics Malaysia). However, based on the income groups, the median of income estimated in this study was comparable to the results from the household survey by DOSM as shown in Table 5.1.

Table 5.1 Comparison of median of income

Income group	Current study 2016	DOSM 2016
T20	RM 12 707	RM 13 148
M40	RM 5502	RM 6275
B40	RM 2140	RM 3000

The discrepancy between the findings from this study and the results from the DOSM surveys could be due to the methodology of data collection. In this study the single question approach was used, by asking the respondent the estimated monthly household income, which in effect led to the possible under-estimation of the household income. The respondents in this study were female breast cancer patients. A study has shown that a single question on the total income in the household and asked to only one member of the household could result in under-reporting compared to over-reporting. Knowledge can be expected to be less for others' income than for one's own (Micklewrigh & Schnepf 2010).

d. Estimated monthly food expenditure

The mean monthly food expenditure was RM 658.51 (333.09, range RM 100.00 - 2000.00). The richer the household the more monthly expenditure they had for food. This finding was comparable to the results of a local study which found that the share of food expenditure increases with increase in income (Yeong-Sheng 2008).

The results in this study show that the percentage of food expenditure from the total household income was relatively smaller in richer household; compared to poorer households. This meant that although the richer households spent more on food, the proportion of this expenditure from the total household income was smaller; whereas the poorer household spent small amount on food, but that expenditure comprised of a large proportion of their household income. This finding is consistent with "Engel's law" which states that the share of household expenditure on food typically falls as income and expenditure increase.

The mean percentage of food expenditure from estimated monthly household income in this study was 20.1% (12.36). This value was comparable to that of the Household Expenditure Survey (HES) in 2014 which was 18.9% and 18.0% in 2016 (Department of Statistics Malaysia).

e. Estimated monthly capacity-to-pay

The median monthly household capacity-to-pay for all respondents was RM 2700 (IQR 1500, 5100). The mean percentage of capacity-to-pay from estimated monthly household income in this study was 80.0% (12.40). This value was comparable to that of the Household Expenditure Survey (HES) in 2014 which was 81.1% and 82.0% in 2016 (Department of Statistics Malaysia).

f. Estimated monthly allopathic treatment expenditure

Approximately 26% (n=88), of the respondents had no monthly treatment expenditure, due to the receiving full financial aids; while for the remainder of the respondents, the estimated median treatment monthly expenditure was RM 112.00 (IQR 72.05, 245.90). This result translated into an estimated median treatment monthly expenditure being 3.4% of the median monthly household income. This finding was slight lower than those found in a review of studies where mean expenditures on chronic diseases ranged from 5% to 59% of household income, household total health expenditure, and household non-food expenditure (Kankeu, et al. 2013).

g. Estimated monthly TCM expenditure

Approximately 73% (n = 239), of the respondents had no monthly TCM expenditure; while for the remainder of the respondents (27%, f=90), the median TCM monthly expenditure was RM 112.00 (IQR 61.00, 250.00). The prevalence of use of TCM in this current study was lower than that of other local studies among breast cancer patients (34.8%, 42.9% and 49.2%), a Canadian study (47%) and an Australian study (87.5%) (Farooqui et al. 2016; Helyer et al. 2006; Kremser et al. 2008; Zulkipli et al. 2017). The differences in prevalence could be due to a difference of study instrument (interview versus self-administered mailed data collection form), differences in the classification of TCM (for example the inclusion of the use of prayer-for-health) and the study sample. In terms of expenditure for TCM there seemed to be a paucity in such studies in Malaysia. One study found that 42.3% of their respondents (of various cancer types) had spent up to RM100 per month (17.3% spent < RM50, while 25% spent RM50-100 per month) (Faraquooi et al. 2016)

h. **Estimated travel and meal expenditures**

The median travel and meals monthly expenditure was RM 90.00 (IQR 49.00, 146.00). This expenditure translated into 7.2% of the estimated mean household income. This finding was like the study in the United States of America among breast cancer patients where non-medical expenditure including travel and meals was 6% of the household income (Arozullah et al. 2004).

i. **Estimated total combined OOP expenditure**

The results of this study showed that the median monthly combined OOP expenditure was RM 237.30 (IQR 138.00, 396.00) per month. Almost half (47.26%) of this expenditure was for allopathic treatment expenditure. In this study the estimated total median out-of-pocket expenditure was statistically significantly different between the income groups: highest in the M40 group, followed by the T20 group and the B40 group. The higher OOP health expenditure among the middle-income group compared to the highest income group in this study could be due to several factors. The results showed that the middle-income respondents had higher OOP expenditure on TCM, travel and food compared to the other income groups. The OOP expenditure on allopathic treatment in the middle-income group was only about RM 30.00 more than the other groups (RM 138.00 among M40 versus RM 109.00 among B40 and RM 101.00 among T20).

The findings in this study in terms of OOP expenditure according to income groups differed from other studies globally which showed that the OOP expenditure increased according to the level of family income (da Silva et al. 2015; Habicht, et al. 2006; Lauzier et al. 2013). Nonetheless, the context of each of these studies needs to be carefully considered before any direct comparisons can be made. This is because the highest expenditure incurred among the M40 respondents was on TCM, not on allopathic medicine, which ultimately resulted in their higher overall OOP expenditure. The reasons why the M40 respondents spent so much on TCM despite their economic constraints need to be explored further.

5.6 Catastrophic Health expenditure

In this study, catastrophic health expenditure (CHE) was defined as spending 40% or more of capacity-to-pay on based on Wagstaff and van Doorslaer (2003). The monthly estimated median combined OOP expenditure for breast cancer was divided by the estimated median household's monthly capacity-to-pay. In this study, the number of households which experienced CHE was 24 (7.3%). This translated into financial protection coverage of 92.7%.

The prevalence of CHE in this study was lower than that captured by the landmark ACTION study, which was 48% for all cancers and 60% for breast cancer in ASEAN countries, a study in Korea found prevalence of CHE was 39.8% while a study Iran found CHE prevalence of 67.9% among cancer patients (Choi et al. 2014; Delavari, Keshtkaran & Setoudehzadeh 2014). This marked difference may be due to the difference in methodology, sample population, study sites and the cushioning effect of the financial aids and thresholds used for CHE and impoverishment.

As for methodology, this current study was retrospective while the ACTION study was prospective. Prospective study may be able to capture more events occurring to the individual patients hence more expenditure data and there may be less or no recall bias.

The ACTION study respondents comprised of cancer patients from low to low-middle income countries of ASEAN; as opposed to Malaysia being a high-middle income country. The higher income per capita in Malaysia could contribute lower prevalence of CHE. Moreover, most of the countries in the ACTION study rely on OOP and private health insurance (WHO 2010a). On the contrary, the health financing system in Malaysia was generally tax-based and highly subsidized. The private or OOP health expenditure in Malaysia was lower than the countries in the ACTION study.

In terms of study sites, a recent prospective study of colorectal cancer patients who received treatment at a local university hospital found that that 47.8% of patients' families experienced CHE (Azzani et al. 2017). As this current study's study sites were all government facilities and one public teaching hospital, the respondents had either zero treatment expenditure or highly subsidized treatment expenditure. Therefore, this could have contributed to the lower CHE prevalence.

The low incidence and prevalence of CHE in this study could also be due to the cushioning effect of the financial safety net. This finding is similar studies in Bangladesh and India where households were able to avoid catastrophic spending because they relied on the availability of informal credit, donations from relatives and selling assets: the richest households relied on income and savings, whereas the poorest households relied more on loans and donations (Hoque, et al. 2015; Rajpal, Kumar & Joe 2018).

Different definitions of CHE could also lead to differences in CHE incidence. Some studies used a threshold OOP share of total household expenditure; others of household 'capacity-to-pay'; or of 'non-food expenditure'. In addition, the threshold used also varies, ranging from 10% to 40%. Also, the CHE calculation in the ACTION study was based on 30% of household income, whereas CHE calculation in this study was based on 40% of capacity-to-pay.

5.7 Impoverishment

In this study, impoverishment was defined as households whose income falls under the poverty line when their OOP for health was deducted from their income. The 2014 national poverty line of RM 930.00 was used.

In this study, the overall headcount for impoverishment was 31 households (9.12%). This meant that impoverishment coverage was approximately 90.88%. If looked at in more detail, the OOP expenditure on breast cancer had actually increased the headcount of poor households from 13 to 31, which was an increase of 138.5%. The relative impact was even greater on the measured poverty gap which was a 25.9% percent increase.

This meant that in this current study the number of households below the poverty line had increased 1.3 times more because of expenditure on breast cancer, and that health expenditure adds another quarter to the pre-payment poverty gap.

As with CHE, there were no known studies on the impoverishing effect of breast cancer treatment which could be compared with the findings of this study. However, there are several studies on impoverishment due to OOP expenditure on general health care. For example, a study in India showed that overall poverty increment after accounting for OOP expenditure was 3.2%, while in China between 9.2% and 23.3% of households were impoverished by medical expenses (Cao, Wang & Wang 2009; Dummer & Cook 2007; Garg & Karan 2008; Li et al. 2012).

5.8 Factors Associated with CHE and Impoverishment Among Breast Cancer Patients

In this study, factors statistically significantly associated with CHE were ethnicity, education level, marital status, household type, location of residence, income and capacity to pay. There were higher proportions of CHE among the following groups: non-Malays, education up to secondary level, not/never married, lived in non-nuclear households, lived in the non-central region compared to those who lived within the central region, the B40 income group and among those whose capacity to pay was less than RM2700.

Ethnicity was associated with CHE in this study. Of the three ethnic groups in this study, the Chinese had the most prevalent of CHE. The Chinese respondents in this study who experienced CHE had low estimated monthly income, low capacity-to-pay, did not have adequate financial aid and had used TCM. They lived within the central region and their stages of cancer were mostly in the not metastatic.

Education level was also found to be associated with CHE in this study, where the respondents whose highest education level was up to the secondary school level had higher prevalence of CHE. Studies found that lower education including illiteracy increases the possibility patients have weaker occupational conditions; hence lower income and capacity-to-pay (Kumar et al. 2015; Moradi et al. 2017; Ramachandran & Jha 2013). However, the findings of other studies need to be considered with caution when comparing them with this current study because those studies were referring to the educational level of the heads of the households; whereas in this study the education level of the respondents was determined. The reasons for this discrepancy of the variables were because the other studies used population data where the head of the households were interviewed, while in this current study the respondents were breast cancer patients who may or may not be the head of the households. Moreover, due to the circumstances in which the data collection was conducted (among breast cancer patients undergoing treatment), the number of personal questions had to be limited to the ones concerning the respondents and not so much of the family. Household types of the respondents also varied with some living with extended family members or even friends where the determination of the household head was problematic let alone determining the level of education of the household head.

Marital status was found to be associated with CHE in this study. The prevalence of CHE was higher among the respondents who were not/never married compared to those who were. This finding could be since a single woman or a widow, would most likely live alone and may not have a large household income. If they were living with the other people, there would most likely be higher household income as the other household members may be earning money, however the capacity-to-pay may be low, as the food expenditure would be higher due to the increased number of household members.

Household type was found to be associated with CHE in this study. The prevalence of CHE was higher among the respondents whose household type was the non-nuclear family compared to nuclear family. This finding could be since a nuclear household would usually be of a smaller size that the non-nuclear family, the income-earner/ head of the household role was clear and most likely the household income would be used solely for the members of this family. On the contrary, in a non-nuclear household, the income earners/ head of the household may not be very clear, and household income may not necessarily be used collectively for the household. Additionally, among the respondents who stayed in a non-nuclear household, there could be an underestimate of the household income as they could not accurately provide information on the income of the head of their households who could be an in-law, siblings or friends.

Household location was associated with CHE in this study, whereby higher proportion of respondents who lived outside of the central region experienced CHE compared to those who lived in the central region. This situation was as expected because most of the medical facilities which provide cancer treatment were in the central region. The farther away the location of the residence of the respondents, the more expenditure incurred for petrol consumption for the vehicles or transportation care. Individuals who experience long commute may also spend more on food while on route. The longer commute also meant there was a higher chance of having to pay toll at the highway, to and from home.

Household income was associated with CHE in this study, whereby higher household income had lower prevalence of CHE compared to lower household income. This was also the finding with household capacity-to-pay. This inverse association between the level of income and capacity-to-pay with the prevalence of CHE has been shown in several studies (Cleopatra & Eunice 2018; Kumar et al. 2015). High household income would allow for more capacity-to-pay and hence less occurrence of CHE. Additionally, higher income household usually purchase medical insurance premiums for extra financial coverage. OOP's share as a percentage of capacity-to-pay is lower among households in which at least one member has health insurance in India (Kumar et al. 2015). Therefore, for high income households not only to they have more disposable income to pay OOP for medical needs, they also have private insurance coverage. The contrary is true for the lower income households.

Other studies on CHE among cancer patients revealed slightly different results. A study among cancer patients in Vietnam revealed that the rates of catastrophic expenditure and impoverishment due to treatment costs for cancer were higher among patients who were 44–60 years old; did not have health insurance; suffered from breast cancer; had cancer stage II; and received multiple treatments Hoang et al. (2017). At regional level, the ACTION study found that having a below-average income, having no health insurance, not having paid work and having attended not higher than primary education, was all associated with higher odds of experiencing catastrophic expenditure (ACTION Study Group 2015).

Health insurance or financial aid was not found to be statistically significant to the prevalence of CHE or impoverishment in this current study. Studies in other countries on the association of health insurance with CHE and impoverishment showed mixed results. In China, it was found that health insurance was a significant determinant of CHE (Yang et al. 2016). On the contrary, a study in Vietnam showed that health insurance had no statistically significant impacts on financial difficulties due to cancer treatment (Hoang et al, 2017). Similarly, the ACTION study also found that in the ASEAN region, the relationship between health insurance and financial catastrophe was not particularly (ACTION Study Group 2015).

As for impoverishment in this study, the factors statistically significantly associated with impoverishment were age, ethnicity, education, employment, location of residence, income and capacity to pay.

Age was associated with impoverishment in this study. The odds of incurring catastrophic expenditure rise have been shown to rise with age. A study in Kenya found that one year raise in an individual's age raises the odds of incurring catastrophic expenditure by 1.16%. This may be explained by the fact that as a person ages, the level of health reduces, making him or her more prone to diseases and more so to NCDs (Mwai & Muriithi 2016).

Ethnicity was also associated with impoverishment in this study. The Chinese ethnic group in this study has the highest prevalent of impoverishment as with CHE discussed earlier. Education level too was associated with impoverishment in this study, where the prevalent of impoverishment were higher among the respondents with lower education level, as was the case with CHE.

Location of respondents was associated with impoverishment in this study whereby respondents whose hometowns were outside the central region and had lodged in family or friends' houses had the highest prevalent of impoverishment. The association between location of respondents' residences and treatment facilities has been shown to cause financial constraints in many studies (Delavari, Keshtkaran, Setoudehzade 2014; Timmons et al. 2009).

Employment was also associated with impoverishment in this study. In this current study the employment status of the respondent, not which of the head of the household was determined. A study found that most cancer patients who are working at the time of their diagnosis experienced a drop in their income and the self-employed can be particularly badly affected (Timmons et al. 2009). A study in Korea found that if a change in economic status results from a change in job status for head of household (job loss), these households are more likely to incur catastrophic health expenditure than households who have not experienced a change in job status (odds ratios 2.17 and 2.63, respectively) (Choi et al. 2014).

5.9 Predictive Factors of CHE and Impoverishment

In this study, two predicting factors for experiencing CHE and impoverishment were ethnicity and location of residence. In this study the non-Malays have higher odds of experiencing financial hardship. This may be due to non-Malay respondents had less access to formal financial aid such as the civil servant health benefits which is a privilege enjoyed by civil servants. With this health benefit, most if not all medical bills for treatment received at government hospitals are waived. The majority of civil servants are of the Malay ethnicity. According to the Prime Minister's Department as of December 2014, civil servants of Chinese ethnicity only made up about 5.2% (Anon. 2015b). Not being a civil servant meant that they were not able to access the free or heavily subsidized health services a civil servant had. Some of these respondents had health insurance but had reached the limit of their insurance claims. Consequently, these factors may have led them to continue treatment at the study sites using OOP expenditure.

The results in this study found that location of residence was a predictive factor for CHE and impoverishment. This finding is like several other studies (Loganathan, Deshmukh, & Raut, 2017; Shukla et al. 2015). The possible factors that could explain why location of residence was a predictive factor for impoverishment. Breast cancer treatment requires patients to travel multiple times to the hospital for interventions, diagnostic procedures, follow up consultations and the like especially during the phase of active treatment. For example, chemotherapy in Malaysia for breast cancer on usually requires 12 cycles, which would mean one or more visits to the hospital per cycle because some chemotherapy requires the patient to have a pre-treatment blood test. In addition to the multiple trips to the hospital, the modes of transportation used were usually by car, as opposed to public transportation. This is because the weak physical condition of the patient would necessitate the use of a car, especially after treatment such as chemotherapy or radiotherapy. Travelling by car, be it a private car or a taxi would be much costlier than travelling by other means of transportation, except for air travel. Travelling by car would incur not only expenditure for fuel but also toll and food.

5.10 UHC Index of Breast Cancer Management

The composite index score for UHC for breast cancer in this current study is 54. The index score was not very high most likely because of the low service coverage of prevention activity (mammogram). The coverage was only about 4% in this study. This low coverage score of mammogram screening may have caused the overall lowering of the UHC index score; as the coverage scores of the other indicators were high. Nonetheless the low mammogram coverage detected by this study was expected because at the national level the coverage was equally low (Aidalina & Syed 2018).

Another study which used the same composite index concept for the monitoring of UHC was published as a World Bank Group's policy research paper (Wagstaff et al. 2016). However, although this current study and the study by Wagstaff et al. (2016) have some similarities in terms of the basic and composite index frameworks, both studies differ in many aspects. The study by Wagstaff et al. (2016) is briefly discussed below for comparison and to illustrate how the results of the UHC index are presented.

The study by Wagstaff et al. (2016) was conducted among 24 Universal Health Coverage Study Series (UNICO) countries. The countries were: Argentina, Brazil, Chile, China, Columbia, Costa Rica, Ethiopia, Georgia, Ghana, Guatemala, India, Indonesia, Jamaica, Kenya, Kyrgyz Republic, Mexico, Nigeria, Peru, Philippines, South Africa, Thailand, Tunisia, Turkey and Vietnam. The indicators for prevention domain used in this study were: 1) four or more antenatal care (ANC) visits; 2) full immunization of a child; 3) breast cancer screening; and 4) cervical cancer screening. The indicators were of simple coverage rather than effective coverage. For treatment domain, the indicators were: 1) whether a baby was delivered by a skilled birth attendant (SBA); 2) whether a child with diarrhoea received given Oral rehydration salts (ORS) or a home-made solution; and 3) whether a child with acute respiratory infection (ARI) received medical treatment and 4) whether or not someone has been admitted to hospital in the previous year. For catastrophic health expenditure, the threshold used was 25% of total consumption and a poverty line of $2.00-a-day for the impoverishment indicator. The chart (Figure 5.1) sourced from Wagstaff et al. (2016) shows the curves which are contours of UHC attainment. The year against the country's name is the average of the years of the surveys from which the data come: for example, if half the indicators were from 2005, and half were from 2007, the year indicated against the country's name was 2006. The countries which had UHC index score of 70 or more were Peru, Philippines, South Africa, Mexico and Costa Rica.

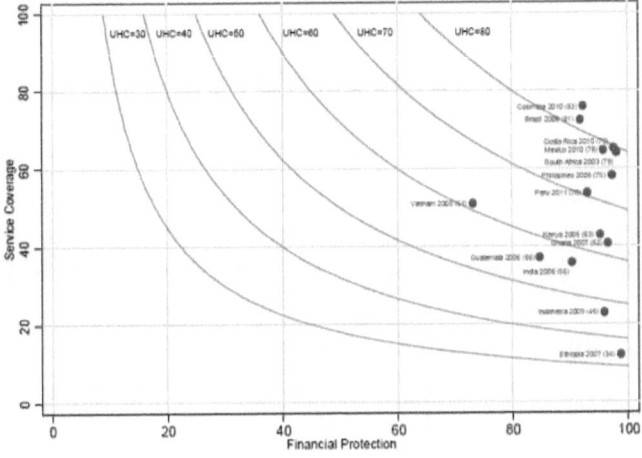

Figure 5.1 Financial protection, service coverage, and UHC index values

In their study, Wagstaff et al. (2016) found a cluster of high-performing countries with UHC scores of between 79 and 84 (Brazil, Colombia, Costa Rica, Mexico, and South Africa) and a cluster of low-performing countries with UHC scores in the range 35–57 (Ethiopia, Guatemala, India, Indonesia, and Vietnam).

Therefore, if based on this classification by Wagstaff et al. (2016), the UHC of breast cancer management in Malaysia according to this current study was approximately in the higher end of the low-performing countries. Because this current study focused on the management of breast cancer, an illness which required specialized and expensive interventions, unlike the illnesses assessed by Wagstaff et al, the UHC index score of 54 could be regarded as modest.

Nonetheless, as this current study was one of the earlier studies on UHC conducted in the year 2015-2016, comparison with other UHC indices was not entirely possible. The UHC index in this study shall be regarded the baseline value against which future results could be compared. Repeated study would give the trend of attainment of UHC in breast cancer management in Malaysia, with the aim of reaching a score of 100% by the year 2030.

5.11 Overall Results Interpretation

In general, the UHC index score measures the combined scores for service coverage and financial protection coverage or the outcome factors in the UHC monitoring theoretical conceptual framework developed by the World Health Organization and the World Bank Group and many other UHC experts.

In terms of the building blocks of the health system, this current study found that the leadership and governance were good. The necessary plans, goals and strategies were available. Relevant documents were also available. A review of the health systems financing showed that the overall health care expenditure of Malaysia was still within the range set by global standards.

Health information system, in terms of publication and availability of vital reports, was found to be good. As for access to essential medicines, in general the access was good as most of the chemotherapy medications were available. There were several medications listed in the WHO list but was not available in the national drug formulary. The more specialized and newer drugs such as targeted therapy were available in the government health facilities' formulary but its use in these facilities was subject to the availability of the medicine and budget. Service delivery needed improvement. There was a limited number of cancer facilities and these facilities were unevenly distributed favoring the urban areas. As for workforce, there were no specific guides as to the number of medical specialists and allied health professionals per specific number of populations in the treatment of cancer, therefore comments could not be made on the currently available number of these specialists.

In this study, the service coverage referred to effective service coverage. As suggested by available literature, effective service coverage is more suitable in assessing coverage of services/interventions in the case of non-communicable diseases, because effective service coverage measures the need of the services and the quality of the services as opposed to merely utilization of services that has been measured by service coverage. The effective service coverage scores in this study were high - between 86 - 100%, except for mammogram screening (4.0 %).

The high effective service coverage score means that a high majority of patients who needed the services (i.e. medical intervention such as chemotherapy), had received the services in a timely manner (timeliness is an important aspect of quality in cancer care as delayed therapy may result in poorer outcome). However, this coverage was restricted to: 1) patients who sought and agreed to receive the services, and 2) patients who were adequately diagnosed and thus deemed needing the service. This effective service coverage score did not consider patients who did not present at medical facilities, either because they did not know they had the disease or because of refusal to get treatment. Hence the effective coverage score only tells us that for those patients who did seek medical help/treatment, a high proportion of them received the services/treatment they needed and of good quality.

In terms of financial protection coverage, the OOP expenditure included in this study were that on health services and intervention the respondents received, travelling and TCM use. Therefore, comparison with other studies on should consider of these expenditures. Financial protection coverage scores in this study were also noted to be high. Prevalence of catastrophic health expenditure was only 7% and prevalence of impoverishment was 9%. The incidence of impoverishment was approximately 5%, as half of the respondents were already in the poor category even before making OOP expenditure for breast cancer. The high financial protection coverage in this study was due to the availability of financial aids, which were civil servant medical benefits, private medical insurance, financial aids from family members and savings. Therefore, the expenditure for health care per se was lower than for travelling and TCM use.

In summary, in the context of this current study, the extent of UHC for breast cancer management in Malaysia is modest with the achievement of UHC composite index score of 55. This index was not meant to be an absolute or one-off value for UHC, but it was meant to be one of a series of UHC indices monitored over time to detect any improvement. However, the improvement has come from increases in receipt of key health interventions, not from reductions in the incidence of out-of-pocket payments on welfare (Wagstaff et al. 2016).

5.12 Limitations of this Study

5.12.1 Study design

The first part of the study involved reviewing the publicly available database and records which contain information on the building blocks of the health system in Malaysia. However, due to some unavoidable administrative constraints, some of the data were not able to be retrieved such as data from the private health care facilities and data on human resource. Hence data of the private health facilities were estimated based on the available information of the facilities' websites while data on human resource were estimated by calculation by the researchers based on available formulas.

The second part of this study was a cross-sectional study. Ideally the study design for assessing the UHC would be a nationwide cohort study. The cohort should be followed from the day of diagnosis for a pre-determined length of time, regardless of where (the type of facility) they sought treatment. The cross-sectional study design was used in this study because it was the most suitable considering the duration of the illness and its treatment as well as the health care-seeking behaviour of Malaysians.

The duration of active treatment for breast cancer is long and may take up to at least 18 months from diagnosis to the completion of targeted therapy. Additionally, in Malaysia, breast cancer patients in Malaysia do not necessarily seek treatment in one health facility throughout their entire course of treatment. There may be crossover of patients between the private and the public hospitals (Lim et al, 2014; Ng et al. 2016). This crossing over or changes in health care providers can make patient follow-up throughout their entire course of treatment almost impossible. An alternative approach was to conduct a cohort study in one facility. However, restricting the cohort in just one facility would result in measuring the UHC based on the performance and expenditure of only that facility. This then would be a misrepresentation of the actual situation in the country because not all cancer facilities provide all services or interventions in one premise and not all cancer patients visit only one cancer care facility throughout their treatment period.

5.12.2 Study location

This current study was carried out in the central region of the country, in the proximity of Kuala Lumpur, the capital city of Malaysia. Ideally the study should include other parts of the country. The rationale for purposively selecting the study sites in this study were as follows.

Firstly, these hospitals were hospitals with resident oncology specialists and radiation oncology facilities. The current epidemiology of breast cancer in this country shows that breast cancer cases are diagnosed at the later stages (Stages III and IV) and thus require breast conserving surgery and/or mastectomy, chemotherapy and radiotherapy. Therefore, most breast cancer cases were expected to ultimately obtain treatment in hospitals such as these four hospitals. Secondly, the selected hospitals were referral hospitals and they serve not only the population in their locality but also from other states. They also receive referrals from the private hospitals. Lastly, the study sites were merely avenues for data collection and the performance of these study locations was not directly assessed. The results captured by this study represented the performance of the whole health system in Malaysia in breast cancer management and not the performance of study locations per se.

The selection of hospitals in the central region as opposed to nationwide in this study would not affect the effective service coverage. The effective service coverage would be the same because all hospitals providing cancer care must adhere to the same SOPs and standards. This finding was reflected in the results of the study by Lim et al. (2014) which was carried out in several hospitals nationwide; and their results were similar to this study's results. Additionally, as mentioned earlier, the fact that the selected facilities were referral hospitals, and they received patients from other parts of the country, could have addressed part of the travel expenditure aspect of the data.

5.12.3 Study population

In this study, the respondents were recruited from the oncology day care facility only and not the wards or at the radiotherapy units. The oncology day care facility was selected because the patients comprised of patients at all stages of cancer and were more clinically comfortable hence could provide better response to interview questions compared to patients in other locations (wards/radiotherapy units).

As this study was conducted in government hospitals, patients treated in private hospitals were under-represented. Public facilities typically involve less OOP health spending than private facilities since public facilities services are subsidized. Therefore, this under-representation of the private health sector utilization may have contributed to a much lower estimate of the level of financial protection coverage, because private hospitals have often been observed to generate the highest OOP expenses especially when medical insurance is unavailable. For example, OOP expenditures associated with a single hospital stay in a private facility for cancer or heart disease in India accounted for between 80-90% of annual per capita household income compared to 40%-50% of annual per capita income for care obtained at a public facility (Alam & Mahal 2014). An analysis for Thailand also concluded that households using inpatient services from private hospitals are more likely to face impoverishment due to OOP spending (Limwattananon, Tangcharoensathien & Prakongsai 2007). On the other hand, although health care services are expensive, private facilities tend to attract patients with higher income and/or having health insurance. Hence the overall effect on OOP may not have be too substantial.

Lastly, as this study was a hospital-based study, individuals who did not seek hospital treatment due to geographical isolation, poverty, or socio-cultural barriers were not included.

5.12.4 Data collection methods

Data collection for service coverage in this study was conducted as retrospective review of the medical records. The rationale of this approach was: the duration of the study was long and due to the time constraint prospective approach was not suitable; the health-seeking behaviour of Malaysian patients as described earlier also made the prospective data collection almost impossible; and lastly the study sites were the final facilities of treatment for most of the patients, the medical records could provide the summary of most of not all the treatment that the respondents had undergone.

Data collection for financial protection coverage was also conducted retrospectively in this study. The rationale was because it was the most feasible option based on the nature of the illness and the constraints in resources. Existing literature show there are no evidence on the optimal survey design in collecting data on health spending (WHO 2011). Prospective data collection usually involves the use of expenditure diary. The use of expenditure diary is good if the health event is brief and if the respondents were highly motivated. Studies have shown that in the case of chronic diseases the quality of diary entry declines as the duration of illness becomes longer (ref. required), as was postulated to occur in this study. On the other hand, retrospective data collection requires the respondent to recall the information (six months for outpatient and up to one year for inpatient events). This latter method was deemed more suitable for this current study.

In this study, only data on household income was collected, while data on wealth was not collected. This was to ensure the length of the data collection interview was acceptable for the respondents. A too-detailed session would make the respondents feel drained and uninterested, resulting in poor engagement thus poor-quality data. Nonetheless, the researchers acknowledge that data on wealth is a better indicator as it represents an accumulated stock rather than a passing flow of resources. Families receiving similar income can experience a different level of economic wellbeing depending on assets that they have (Wolff 1998). The income sourced from assets such as financial investments or real estate rentals could support consumption and living, even if the owner is not employed. On the other hand, many families have zero or negative net worth despite having a regular income above the poverty line (Khalid 2011).

The literatures suggest that patients tend to underreport their use of health care resources and therefore the costs reported in this study may be in the lower bound (Evans & Crawford 1999; Longo & Bereza 2011; Roberts et al 1996). This was especially so in cases where the respondents were unemployed elderly women who lived in an extended family household. A study on the challenges of eliciting income and other socioeconomic data from face-to-face interview showed similar findings; where propensity to not report income was also found to increase with age the respondents (Turrell 2000). To overcome this uncertainty, the respondents in this study were asked about the occupation of the heads of the households so that their household income could be estimated. Other challenges in eliciting income data such as recall bias and the interview process being taxing were like the ones extensively discussed by Moore & Welniak (2000) in their review of literature and thus, were limitations of this study.

Apart from underestimation of income, there may be an under estimation of expenditure. In this study the expenditure data was based on what was reported by the respondents and were not verified objectively. The reported OOP expenditure could have been cross-checked with the medical records for a higher degree of accuracy. Also, the OOP expenditure of terminally ill patients was not included in this study. This category of patients may incur high OOP expenditure. Secondly, the sum of OOP expenditure for allopathic treatment used in the calculations was net of financial aids. Moreover, there may have been reporting bias in the use of TCM because the respondents may not want to disclose their usage. To overcome this reluctance of disclosure, the interview technique used was as non-intimidating as possible to ensure the respondents were relaxed and forthcoming. The inclusion of expenditure net of financial aid was representing the actual scenario of breast cancer patients while the non-inclusion of the terminally ill patients was a limitation of this study.

5.12.5 Study results

The study results were analysed based on the available frameworks and analytical processes available in the years 2015 and 2016. As discussions on UHC monitoring and evaluation is ongoing globally, any frameworks or analytical processes beyond the year 2016 were not taken into consideration in this study. Comparisons of findings of this study with the other UHC studies contexts should be done with caution because of the differences in context, definition and methods of calculation

5.13 Strengths of This Study

The framework, set of indicators and targets for measuring UHC in breast cancer management were developed based on the adoption of available literature on UHC, prior to and during the study period. To date and to the researchers' knowledge, the combination of framework, indicators and targets for UHC of breast cancer used in this study was the first of its kind and they encompassed the whole concept of UHC as opposed to fragments of UHC.

In this current study, all indicators used were evidence-based clinical guidelines which have been converted into quality performance indicators, which were then converted into UHC indicators. Again, as to the researchers' knowledge, this approach was the first of its kind. In general, there are no rigid rules on how indicators should be selected. Boerma et al. (2014) had stated that countries should select those indicators that are most relevant to their own situation, if they adhere to the criteria detailed in numerous publications as discussed in Chapter 2 of this thesis. Although there were some concerns of using converting clinical guidelines into performance measures, the potential benefits of performance measures derived from evidence-based guidelines can help improve the quality of medical care (Walter et al. 2004).

As this study is the first of its kind in Malaysia at present, it can be considered a precedent of future research on assessing the extent of UHC, and its findings could be used as baseline data for comparison with future data. This study, if carried out periodically in the following few years, could provide the trend in UHC coverage in breast cancer management in Malaysia, in the country joins the global goal of achieving UHC in the year 2030.

The framework, set of indicators and targets for measuring UHC in breast cancer management were developed based on the adoption of available literature on UHC, prior to and during the study period. To date and to the researchers' knowledge, the combination of framework, indicators and targets for UHC of breast cancer used in this study was the first of its kind and they encompassed the whole concept of UHC as opposed to fragments of UHC.

In this current study, all indicators used were evidence-based clinical guidelines which have been converted into quality performance indicators, which were then converted into UHC indicators. Again, as to the researchers' knowledge, this approach was the first of its kind. In general, there are no rigid rules on how indicators should be selected. Boerma et al. (2014) had stated that countries should select those indicators that are most relevant to their own situation, if they adhere to the criteria detailed in numerous publications as discussed in Chapter 2 of this thesis. Although there were some concerns of using converting clinical guidelines into performance measures, the potential benefits of performance measures derived from evidence-based guidelines can help improve the quality of medical care (Walter et al. 2004).

As this study is the first of its kind in Malaysia at present, it can be considered a precedent of future research on assessing the extent of UHC, and its findings could be used as baseline data for comparison with future data. This study, if carried out periodically in the following few years, could provide the trend in UHC coverage in breast cancer management in Malaysia, in the country joins the global goal of achieving UHC in the year 2030.

VI CONCLUSION AND RECOMMENDATIONS

6.1 Conclusion

Based on this study, the composite index score for Universal Health Coverage for breast cancer management in Malaysia is 54. This index was considered modest based on available studies on UHC. Effective service coverage and financial protection coverage in breast cancer management were also found to be good where there were high levels of service coverage for majority of the services. Two of the services, however, did not fare very well: mammogram screening and use of the drug Trastuzumab which is a targeted therapy for breast cancer. It was also found on this study that there are high levels of financial risk protection, where 91% and 93% of the patients experienced CHE and impoverishment from spending for breast cancer, respectively. Predicting factors for both CHE and impoverishment are ethnicity (being non-Malay) and patients staying outside of the central region of the country.

This study also found that Malaysia has a good set of building blocks of the health system in terms of leadership and governance and health information system. However, for the other health systems building blocks, the country's current achievements need to be improved. For example, private health expenditure is on the rise and if it persists, this can negatively influence the efforts in achieving UHC. There are also inadequacies in service delivery such as human resource and accessibility to essential medicines.

This was a preliminary study on UHC, particularly on breast cancer in Malaysia, and the results were subjected to the study limitations. Nevertheless, it is anticipated that this research may entice many more researches on universal health coverage in Malaysia to be carried out in the future, using the WHO and the WBG definitions, frameworks, indicators and targets; as well as using more advanced and refined methodologies.

6.2 Recommendations for Future Research

The recommendation for future research is as follows. Firstly, studies should be done to determine why non-Malays are more prone to CHE and impoverishment in getting treatment and interventions for breast cancer. Secondly, studies should also be done to further study spatial accessibility of cancer facilities throughout the country, as location of the patients' residences was also a predictive factor for both CHE and impoverishment. Thirdly, as the mammogram screening uptake was low and impacted on the overall UHC index score, further studies need to be done to explore why women still do not undergo mammogram screening despite the promotion, subsidy and availability of mammogram services.

Additionally, it is recommended that the assessment of the extent of UHC of breast cancer such as this current study be carried out every few years to determine the trend in UHC coverage before the year 2030. Because this current study would have provided the baseline data for the years 2015-2016. The assessment should be subsequently conducted every five years after 2020, which will be in the years 2025 and 2030.

Also, as this study was the first known type of study for breast cancer, the frameworks, indicators and targets proposed and used in this study could be further refined based on the available data at the time of the next study. In estimating the OOP expenditure for breast cancer, modelling technique could also be explored. A modelling study on OOP health expenditure at the household level has already been done in Greece (Matsaganis, Mitrakos & Tsakloglou 2009). Also, if data of OOP expenditure for breast cancer was collected from patient interview, cross-checking the data with the patients' medical records or other written records should be done where possible.

6.3 Policy implications based on this study

Based on this study, policy makers could further investigate the financial protection coverage for breast cancer patients particularly among the non-Malay patients and those who live far from treatment facilities, as these two groups of patients are at a higher risk of facing financial difficulties.

Policy makers could also further explore on the challenges faced by Malaysian women which hinder them from undergoing mammogram screening. Based on this study, the uptake of mammogram is about 4 percent only and the low coverage negatively impact the overall UHC index score. New approaches may need to be taken to encourage women to come forth for mammogram screening. Increase in mammogram screening uptake will increase the service coverage score and improve the overall UHC index score. An increase of uptake to about 30% can increase the UHC score to 88, while an increase to about 50% will increase the UHC score to approximately 100.

Additionally, several health systems building blocks may need to be addressed by the policymakers and stakeholders. Human resource in cancer management should be increased as planned in the strategic plans and blueprints. Secondly, the accessibility of essential cancer medicines should be addressed and improved.

References

Accountant General's Department of Malaysia. Travelling allowance. *Treasury Circular* 2/2006.

ACTION Study Group. 2015. Catastrophic health expenditure and 12-month mortality associated with cancer in Southeast Asia: results from a longitudinal study in eight countries. *BMC Medicine* 13(1):190.

Ahmad, B. A., Khairatul, K., & Farnaza, A. 2017. An assessment of patient waiting and consultation time in a primary healthcare clinic. *Malaysian Family Physician: The Official Journal of the Academy of Family Physicians of Malaysia* 12(1):14.

Aidalina, M., & Syed, A. M. 2018. The uptake of Mammogram screening in Malaysia and its associated factors: A systematic review. *The Medical Journal of Malaysia* 73(4): 202-211.

Alam, K., & Mahal, A. 2014. Economic impacts of health shocks on households in low- and middle-income countries: a review of the literature. *Globalization and Health* 10(1):21.

Albert, J. M., & Das, P. 2012). Quality assessment in oncology. *International Journal of Radiation Oncology* Biology* Physics* 83(3):773-781.

American College of Surgeons. NAPBC Standards Manual. 2014. https://www.facs.org/~/media/files/quality%20programs/napbc/2014%20napbc%20standards%20manual.ashx [30 Jun 2015].

Anderson, B.O., Yip, C.H., Smith, R.A., Shyyan, R., Sener, S.F., Eniu, A., Carlson, R.W., Azavedo, E. and Harford, J. 2008. Guideline implementation for breast healthcare in low-income and middle-income countries. *Cancer* 113 (S8):2221-2243.

Anon. 2015a. Jahit baju raya guna kain lama. Sinar Online, 7 July http://www.sinarharian.com.my/edisi/perak/jahit-baju-raya-guna-kain-lama-1.408373 [5 August 2015].

Anon. 2015b. 1.6 juta pegawai perkhidmatan awam sehingga 2014. Kosmo Online, 12 Mac. http://ww1.kosmo.com.my/kosmo/content.asp?y=2015 [21 July 2016].

Anon. 2016a. Saya tak sanggup lihat mak sakit. 31 August. http://pahang-ku.blogspot.com/2016/08/saya-tak-sanggup-lihat-mak-sakit.html [5 September 2016].

Anon. 2016b. Selagi hayat dikandung badan. Sinar Online, 17 May. https://www.sinarharian.com.my [5 September 2016].

Arozullah, A.M., Calhoun, E.A., Wolf, M., Finley, D.K., Fitzner, K.A., Heckinger, E.A., Gorby, N.S., Schumock, G.T. & Bennett, C.L. 2004. The financial burden of cancer: estimates from a study of insured women with breast cancer. *J Support Oncol* 2(3):271-278.

ASCO-NCCN Quality Measures for Breast and Colorectal cancer care. https://www.asco.org/ASCOv2/Practice+&+Guidelines/Quality+Care/Quality+Measurement+&+Improvement/ASCO-NCCN+Quality+Measures

Atun, R., Knaul, & F. M. 2012. Innovative financing: local and global opportunities. Closing the Cancer Divide 2: 255.

Azzani, M., Yahya, A., Roslani, A. C., & Su, T. T. 2017. Catastrophic health expenditure among colorectal cancer patients and families: a case of malaysia. *Asia Pacific Journal of Public Health* 29(6):485-494.

Azizah, A. M., Norsaleha, I. T., Noor Hashimah, A., Asmah, Z. A., & Mastulu, W. 2016. *Malaysian National Cancer Registry Report 2007–2011*. National Cancer Institute.

Backman, G., Hunt, P., Khosla, R., Jaramillo-Strouss, C., Fikre, B.M., Rumble, C., Pevalin, D., Páez, D.A., Pineda, M.A., Frisancho, A. & Tarco, D. 2008. Health systems and the right to health: an assessment of 194 countries. *The Lancet* 372(9655):2047-2085.

Bahagian Kawalan Penyakit Kementerian Kesihatan Malaysia. n.d. MYCDCGP - National Cancer Control Blueprint Master Plan 2008 to 2015.

Bao, H., Yang, F., Wang, X., Su, S., Liu, D., Fu, R., Zhang, H. and Liu, M. 2015. Developing a set of quality indicators for breast cancer care in China. *International Journal for Quality in Health Care* 27(4):291-296.

Benyoussef, A., & Christian, B. 1977. Health care in developing countries. *Social Science & Medicine (1967)*, *11*(6-7), 399-408.

Bennett F. Primary health care and developing countries. 1979. *Soc Sci Med*; 13A: 505-514.

Berry, D.A., Cirrincione, C., Henderson, I.C., Citron, M.L., Budman, D.R., Goldstein, L.J., Martino, S., Perez, E.A., Muss, H.B., Norton, L. and Hudis, C. 2006. Estrogen-receptor status and outcomes of modern chemotherapy for patients with node-positive breast cancer. *JAMA* 295(14):1658-1667.

Bhoo-Pathy, N. 2015. Prioritising strategies to addess the economic impact of cancer in South East Asia. Presented at ESMO Asia.

Bhuvan, K. C., Yusoff, Z. B. M., Alrasheedy, A. A., & Othman, S. 2013. The Characteristics and the Pharmacological Management of Cancer Pain and Its Effect on the Patients' Daily Activities and their Quality of Life: A Cross–Sectional study from Malaysia. *Journal of clinical and diagnostic research: JCDR*, 7(7), 1408.

Boerma, J. T., Bryce, J., Kinfu, Y., Axelson, H., & Victora, C. G. 2008. Mind the gap: equity and trends in coverage of maternal, newborn, and child health services in 54 Countdown countries. *The Lancet* 371(9620):1259-1267.

Boerma, T., AbouZahr, C., Evans, D., & Evans, T. 2014a. Monitoring intervention coverage in the context of universal health coverage. *PLoS Medicine* 11(9): e1001728.

Boerma, T., Eozenou, P., Evans, D., Evans, T., Kieny, M. P., & Wagstaff, A. 2014b. Monitoring progress towards universal health coverage at country and global levels. *PLoS Medicine* 11(9):e1001731.

Boing, A. C., Bertoldi, A. D., Posenato, L. G., & Peres, K. G. 2014. The influence of health expenditures on household impoverishment in Brazil. *Revista de saude publica* 48: 797-807.

Bonadonna, G., Valagussa, P., Zucali, R., & Salvadori, B. 1995. Primary chemotherapy in surgically resectable breast cancer. *CA: A Cancer Journal for Clinicians* 45(4):227-243.

Boo Su-Lyn. 2016. Why new cancer drugs are unavailable in Malaysian public hospitals. Malay Mail, 5 December: https://www.malaymail.com/hy-new-cancer-drugs-are-unavailable-in-malaysian-public-hospitals [3 January 2017].

Buigut, S., Ettarh, R., & Amendah, D. D. 2015. Catastrophic health expenditure and its determinants in Kenya slum communities. *International Journal for Equity in Health* 14(1):46.

Cameron, A., Ewen, M., Ross-Degnan, D., Ball, D. and Laing, R. 2009. Medicine prices, availability, and affordability in 36 developing and middle-income countries: a secondary analysis. *The Lancet* 373(9659):240-249.

Cancer Research UK. 2015. Cancer waiting times definitions by country. https://www.cancerresearchuk.org/ [7 June 2015].

Cao, S., Wang, X., & Wang, G. 2009. Lessons learned from China's fall into the poverty trap. *Journal of Policy Modeling* 31(2):298-307.

Chai, S. T., & Hamid, T. A. 2015. Population ageing and the Malaysian Chinese: Issues and challenges. *Malaysian Journal of Chinese Studies* 4(1):1-13.

Chen, L., Evans, D., Evans, T., Sadana, R., Stilwell, B., Travis, P., van Lerberghe, W. and Zurn, P. 2006. *The World Health Report 2006: Working Together for Health*. Geneva: World Health Organization.

Chen, F., Puig, M., Yermilov, I., Malin, J., Schneider, E.C., Epstein, A.M., Kahn, K.L., Ganz, P.A. and Gibbons, M.M. 2011. Using breast cancer quality indicators in a vulnerable population. *Cancer* 117(15):3311-3321.

Chivukula, M. V., & Tisocki, K. 2018. Approaches to improving access to essential cancer medicines in the WHO South-East Asia Region. *WHO South-East Asia journal of public health*, 7(2), 62.

Choi, J. W., Cho, K. H., Choi, Y., Han, K. T., Kwon, J. A., & Park, E. C. 2014. Changes in economic status of households associated with catastrophic health expenditures for cancer in South Korea. *Asian Pacific Journal of Cancer Prevention* 15(6), 2713-2717.

Chua, H. T., & Cheah, J. C. H. (2012, June). Financing universal coverage in Malaysia: a case study. In *BMC public health* (Vol. 12, No. 1, p. S7). BioMed Central.

Clauser, S. B., Wagner, E. H., Bowles, E. J. A., Tuzzio, L., & Greene, S. M. 2011. Improving modern cancer care through information technology. *American Journal of Preventive Medicine* 40(5):S198-S207.

Cleopatra, I., & Eunice, K. 2018. Household Catastrophic Health Expenditure: Evidence from Nigeria. Microeconomics and Macroeconomics 6(1):1-8.

Clinical Research Center (n.d.). National Healthcare Establishment and Workforce Statistics.http://www.crc.gov.my/nhsi/category/publications/hospital-establishment-workforce [11 July 2015].

Cold, S., Düring, M., Ewertz, M., Knoop, A., & Møller, S. 2005. Does timing of adjuvant chemotherapy influence the prognosis after early breast cancer? Results of the Danish

Breast Cancer Cooperative Group (DBCG). *British Journal of Cancer* 93(6): 627.

da Silva, M. T., Barros, A. J., Bertoldi, A. D., de Andrade Jacinto, P., Matijasevich, A., Santos, I. S., & Tejada, C. A. O. 2015. Determinants of out-of-pocket health expenditure on children: an analysis of the 2004 Pelotas Birth Cohort. *International Journal for Equity in Health*, 141: 53.

Delavari, H., Keshtkaran, A., & Setoudehzadeh, F. 2014. Catastrophic health expenditures and coping strategies in households with cancer patients in Shiraz Namazi hospital. *Middle East Journal of Cancer* 5(1): 13-22.

Department of Statistics Malaysia. Current population estimates, Malaysia 2014-2016. https://www.dosm.gov.my/v1/index.php.

Desch, C.E., McNiff, K.K., Schneider, E.C., Schrag, D., McClure, J., Lepisto, E., Donaldson, M.S., Kahn, K.L., Weeks, J.C., Ko, C.Y. and Stewart, A.K. 2008. American society of clinical oncology/national comprehensive cancer network quality measures. *Journal of Clinical Oncology* 26(21):3631-3637.

Dummer, T. J., & Cook, I. G. 2007. Exploring China's rural health crisis: processes and policy implications. *Health Policy* 83(1):1-16.

Early Breast Cancer Trialists' Collaborative Group. 2008. Adjuvant chemotherapy in oestrogen-receptor-poor breast cancer: patient-level meta-analysis of randomised trials. *The Lancet* 371(9606):29-40.

Early Breast Cancer Trialists' Collaborative Group. 2011. Effect of radiotherapy after breast-conserving surgery on 10-year recurrence and 15-year breast cancer death: meta-analysis of individual patient data for 10 801 women in 17 randomised trials. *The Lancet* 378(9804):1707-1716.

Ebener, S., Roth, S., & Khetrapal, S. (2018). Building Capacity for Geo-Enabling Health Information Systems: Supporting Equitable Health Services and Well-Being For ALL.

Economic Planning Unit. 2018. The Malaysian economy in figures 2018. http://epu.gov.my/sites/default/files/MEIF_2018.pdf [16 January 2018].

Edge, S. B., & Compton, C. C. 2010. The American Joint Committee on Cancer: the 7th edition of the AJCC cancer staging manual and the future of TNM. *Annals of Surgical Oncology* 17(6): 1471-1474.

Eniu, A., Carlson, R.W., El Saghir, N.S., Bines, J., Bese, N.S., Vorobiof, D., Masetti, R., Anderson, B.O. and Breast Health Global Initiative Treatment Panel. 2008. Guideline implementation for breast healthcare in low-and middle-income countries: treatment resource allocation. *Cancer* 113(S8):2269-2281.

European Society of Breast Cancer Specialists (EUSOMA). https://www.eusoma.org/en/guidelines/quality-indicators/ [11 July 2015].

Evans, C., & Crawford, B. 1999. Patient self-reports in pharmacoeconomic studies. *Pharmacoeconomics* 15(3):241-256.

Evans, D. B., Saksena, P., Elovainio, R., & Boerma, T. 2012. *Measuring Progress towards Universal Coverage*. Geneva: World Health Organization.

Ezat, W. P., & Aljunid, S. 2010. Cost-effectiveness of HPV vaccination in the prevention of cervical cancer in Malaysia. *Asian Pac J Cancer Prev* 11(1):79-90.

Fantoni, S. Q., Peugniez, C., Duhamel, A., Skrzypczak, J., Frimat, P., & Leroyer, A. 2010. Factors related to return to work by women with breast cancer in northern France. *Journal of Occupational Rehabilitation* 20(1):49-58.

Farooqui, M., Hassali, M. A., Shatar, A. K. A., Farooqui, M. A., Saleem, F., ul Haq, N., & Othman, C. N. 2016. Use of complementary and alternative medicines among Malaysian cancer patients: A descriptive study. *Journal of Traditional and Complementary Medicine* 6(4):321-326.

Farolfi, A., Scarpi, E., Rocca, A., Mangia, A., Biglia, N., Gianni, L., Tienghi, A., Valerio, M.R., Gasparini, G., Amaducci, L. and Faedi, M. 2015. Time to initiation of adjuvant chemotherapy in patients with rapidly proliferating early breast cancer. *European Journal of Cancer* 51(14):1874-1881.

Fasola, G., Macerelli, M., Follador, A., Rihawi, K., Aprile, G., & Mea, V. D. 2014. Health information technology in oncology practice: a literature review. *Cancer informatics* 13:S12417.

Ferlay, J., Shin, H. R., Bray, F., Forman, D., Mathers, C., & Parkin, D. M. (2010). Estimates of worldwide burden of cancer in 2008: GLOBOCAN 2008. *International Journal of Cancer* 127(12):2893-2917.

Flores, G., Krishnakumar, J., O'donnell, O., & Van Doorslaer, E. 2008. Coping with health-care costs: implications for the measurement of catastrophic expenditures and poverty. *Health Economics* 17(12):1393-1412.

Foley, K. M., Wagner, J. L., Joranson, D. E., & Gelband, H. 2006. Pain control for people with cancer and AIDS. *Disease control priorities in developing countries* 2: 981-994.

Fradelos, E. C., Papathanasiou, I. V., Mitsi, D., Tsaras, K., Kleisiaris, C. F., & Kourkouta, L. 2014. Health based geographic information systems (GIS) and their applications. *Acta Informatica Medica* 22(6):402.

Garg, C. C., & Karan, A. K. 2008. Reducing out-of-pocket expenditures to reduce poverty: a disaggregated analysis at rural-urban and state level in India. *Health policy and planning* 24(2):116-128.

Gralow, J.R., Krakauer, E., Anderson, B.O., Ilbawi, A., Porter, P., Gospodarowicz, M., Feldman, S., Rodriguez-Galindo, C., Frazier, L., Lehmann, L. and Shulman, L. 2012. Core elements for provision of cancer care and control in low- and middle-income countries: 123-65. Cambridge (MA): *Harvard Global Equity Initiative.*

Ghany, D. A. 2013. Impact of adjuvant chemotherapy delay on survival in cancer breast patients. *The Chinese-German Journal of Clinical Oncology* 12(1):20-24.

Gianni, L., Pienkowski, T., Im, Y.H., Roman, L., Tseng, L.M., Liu, M.C., Lluch, A., Staroslawska, E., de la Haba-Rodriguez, J., Im, S.A. and Pedrini, J.L. 2012. Efficacy and safety of neoadjuvant pertuzumab and trastuzumab in women with locally advanced, inflammatory, or early HER2-positive breast cancer (NeoSphere): a randomised multicentre, open-label, phase 2 trial. *The Lancet Oncology* 13(1):25-32.

Glassman, A., & Chalkidou, K. 2012. Priority-setting in health: building institutions for smarter public spending. Washington, DC: Center for Global Development.

Global AIDS Response Progress Report Malaysia 2015.

Gotsadze, G., Zoidze, A., & Rukhadze, N. 2009. Household catastrophic health expenditure: evidence from Georgia and its policy implications. *BMC Health Services Research* 9(1):69.

Govender, V., McIntyre, D., & Loewenson, R. 2008. Progress towards the Abuja target for government spending on health care in East and Southern Africa.

Greenberg, A., Angus, H., Sullivan, T., & Brown, A. D. 2005. Development of a set of strategy-based system-level cancer care performance indicators in Ontario, Canada. *International Journal for Quality in Health Care* 17(2):107-114.

Greer, S. L., & Méndez, C. A. 2015. Universal health coverage: a political struggle and governance challenge. *American Journal of Public Health* 105(S5): S637-S639.

Guy Jr, G.P., Yabroff, K.R., Ekwueme, D.U., Virgo, K.S., Han, X., Banegas, M.P., Soni, A., Zheng, Z., Chawla, N. and Geiger, A.M. 2015. Healthcare expenditure burden among non-elderly cancer survivors, 2008–2012. *American Journal of Preventive Medicine* 49(6): S489-S497.

Haas, S., Hatt, L., Leegwater, A., El-Khoury, M., & Wong, W. 2012. *Indicators for Measuring Universal Health Coverage: A Five-Country Analysis (Draft)*. Bethesda, MD: Health Systems, 20, 20.

Habicht, J., Xu, K., Couffinhal, A., & Kutzin, J. 2006. Detecting changes in financial protection: creating evidence for policy in Estonia. *Health Policy and Planning* 216: 421-431.

Hassett, M. J., O'malley, A. J., & Keating, N. L. 2009. Factors influencing changes in employment among women with newly diagnosed breast cancer. *Cancer* 115(12):2775-2782.

Hazard, H. W., Gorla, S. R., Scholtens, D., Kiel, K., Gradishar, W. J., & Khan, S. A. (2008). Surgical resection of the primary tumor, chest wall control, and survival in women with metastatic breast cancer. *Cancer* 113(8): 011-2019.

Helyer, L.K., Chin, S., Chui, B.K., Fitzgerald, B., Verma, S., Rakovitch, E., Dranitsaris, G. and Clemons, M. 2006. The use of complementary and alternative medicines among patients with locally advanced breast cancer–a descriptive study. *BMC cancer* 6(1):39.

Hoang, V.M., Pham, C.P., Vu, Q.M., Ngo, T.T., Tran, D.H., Bui, D., Pham, X.D., Tran, D.K. and Mai, T.K., 2017. Household Financial Burden and Poverty Impacts of Cancer Treatment in Vietnam. *BioMed Research International* 2017:9350147-9350147.

Hoque, M. E., Dasgupta, S. K., Naznin, E., & Al Mamun, A. 2015. Household coping strategies for delivery and related healthcare cost: findings from rural Bangladesh. *Tropical Medicine & International Health* 20(10):1368-1375.

Hospis Malaysia. 2016. Palliative care needs assessment: Malaysia. https://www.hospismalaysia.org/wp-content/uploads/2016/10/Palliative-Care-Needs-Assessment-Malaysia-2016.pdf [3 Mac 2017].

Hughes, M.E., Ottesen, R., Niland, J.C., Edge, S.B., Theriault, R.L., Wilson, J., Blayney, D.W., Wong, Y. and Weeks, J.C. 2009. Quality of breast cancer care in NCCN centers as assessed by the ASCO/NCCN quality measures: overall performance and reasons for nonconcordance. *Journal of Clinical Oncology* 27(15S):6506-6506.

International Agency for Research on Cancer. 2002. IARC *Handbooks of Cancer Prevention* (Vol. 6). The Agency.

International Agency for Research on Cancer. 2012. *GLOBOCAN 2012: Estimated Cancer Incidence, Mortality and Prevalence Worldwide.*

Ir M, D., Johari Dato Mohd Ghazali, R., Hazilah Abd Manaf, N., Hassan Asaari Abdullah, A., Abu Bakar, A., Salikin, F., Umapathy, M., Ali, R., Bidin, N. and Ismefariana Wan Ismail, W. 2011. Hospital waiting time: the forgotten premise of healthcare service delivery? *International Journal of Health Care Quality Assurance* 24(7):506-522.

Jagsi, R., Hawley, S.T., Abrahamse, P., Li, Y., Janz, N.K., Griggs, J.J., Bradley, C., Graff, J.J., Hamilton, A. and Katz, S.J. 2014. Impact of adjuvant chemotherapy on long-term employment of survivors of early-stage breast cancer. *Cancer* 120(12):1854-1862.

Jain, M., & Mukherjee, K. 2016. Economic burden of breast cancer to the households in Punjab, India. *International Journal of Medicine & Public Health* 6(1).

Jang, H., Baek, J., Nam, K. S., & Kim, S. 2016. Determination of the optimal time for tamoxifen treatment in combination with radiotherapy. *International Journal of Oncology* 49(5):2147-2154.

Jemal, A., Siegel, R., Xu, J., & Ward, E. (2010). Cancer statistics, 2010. *CA: a cancer journal for clinicians*, *60*(5), 277-300.

Jowett, M., Brunal, M. P., Flores, G., & Cylus, J. 2016. Spending targets for health: no magic number.

Kankeu, H. T., Saksena, P., Xu, K., & Evans, D. B. 2013. The financial burden from non-communicable diseases in low- and middle-income countries: a literature review. *Health Research Policy and Systems* 11(1):31.

Khalid, M. A. 2011. Household wealth in Malaysia: Composition and inequality among ethnic groups. *Jurnal Ekonomi Malaysia* 45(1):71-80.

Khoda, L., Kapa, B., Singh, K., Gojendra, T., Singh, L., & Sharma, K. (2015). Evaluation of modified triple test (clinical breast examination, ultrasonography, and fine-needle aspiration cytology) in the diagnosis of palpable breast lumps. *Journal of Medical Society* 29(1): 26-26.

Kimani, D. N., Mugo, M. G., & Kioko, U. M. 2016. Catastrophic health expenditures and impoverishment in Kenya. *European Scientific Journal* 12(15).

Kremser, T.A.A.K.S.A.H., Evans, A., Moore, A., Luxford, K., Begbie, S., Bensoussan, A., Marigliani, R. and Zorbas, H. 2008. Use of complementary therapies by Australian women with breast cancer. *The Breast* 17(4):387-394.

Kumar, K., Singh, A., Kumar, S., Ram, F., Singh, A., Ram, U., Negin, J. and Kowal, P.R., 2015. Socio-economic differentials in impoverishment effects of out-of-pocket health expenditure in China and India: evidence from WHO SAGE. *PloS One* 10(8):p.e0135051.

Kutzin, J. (2008). *Health Financing Policy: A Guide for Decision-Makers*. Health Financing Policy Paper. Copenhagen, WHO Regional Office for Europe, 24.

Lammers, P., Criscitiello, C., Curigliano, G., & Jacobs, I. 2014. Barriers to the use of trastuzumab for HER2+ breast cancer and the potential impact of biosimilars: a physician survey in the United States and emerging markets. *Pharmaceuticals* 7(9):943-953.

Laronga, C., Gray, J.E., Siegel, E.M., Lee, J.H., Fulp, W.J., Fletcher, M., Schreiber, F., Brown, R., Levine, R.,

Cartwright, T. and Abesada-Terk Jr, G. 2014. Florida initiative for quality cancer care: improvements in breast cancer quality indicators during a 3-year interval. *Journal of the American College of Surgeons* 219(4):638-645.

Lauby-Secretan, B., Scoccianti, C., Loomis, D., Benbrahim-Tallaa, L., Bouvard, V., Bianchini, F., & Straif, K. 2015. Breast-cancer screening—viewpoint of the IARC Working Group. *New England Journal of Medicine* 372(24): 2353-58.

Lauzier, S., Lévesque, P., Mondor, M., Drolet, M., Coyle, D., Brisson, J., Mâsse, B., Provencher, L., Robidoux, A. and Maunsell, E. 2013. Out-of-pocket costs in the year after early breast cancer among Canadian women and spouses. *Journal of the National Cancer Institute* 105(4):280-292.

Leong, S.P., Shen, Z.Z., Liu, T.J., Agarwal, G., Tajima, T., Paik, N.S., Sandelin, K., Derossis, A., Cody, H. and Foulkes, W.D. 2010. Is breast cancer the same disease in Asian and Western countries? *World Journal of Surgery* 34(10):2308-2324.

Levine, M., & Steering Committee on Clinical Practice Guidelines for the Care and Treatment of Breast Cancer. 2001. Clinical practice guidelines for the care and treatment of breast cancer: adjuvant systemic therapy for node-positive breast cancer (summary of the 2001 update). *Canadian Medical Association Journal* 164(5):644-646.

Li, Wen-Fei, Ying Sun, Yan-Ping Mao, Lei Chen, Yuan-Yuan Chen, Mo Chen, Li-Zhi Liu, Ai-Hua Lin, Li Li, and Jun Ma. 2013. Proposed lymph node staging system using the International Consensus Guidelines for lymph node levels is predictive for nasopharyngeal carcinoma patients from endemic areas treated with intensity modulated radiation therapy. *International Journal of Radiation Oncology* Biology* Physics* 86(2): 249-256.

Li, Y., Wu, Q., Xu, L., Legge, D., Hao, Y., Gao, L., Ning, N. and Wan, G. 2012. Factors affecting catastrophic health expenditure and impoverishment from medical expenses in China: policy implications of universal health insurance. *Bulletin of the World Health Organization* 90:664-671.

Lim, G.C., Aina, E.N., Cheah, S.K., Ismail, F., Ho, G.F., Tho, L.M., Yip, C.H., Taib, N.A., Chong, K.J., Dharmaratnam, J. and Abdullah, M.M. 2014. Closing the global cancer divide-performance of breast cancer care services in a middle-income developing country. *BMC Cancer* 14(1):212.

Limwattananon, S., Tangcharoensathien, V., & Prakongsai, P. 2007. Catastrophic and poverty impacts of health payments: results from national household surveys in Thailand. *Bulletin of the World Health Organization* 85:600-606.

Loganathan, K., Deshmukh, P. R., & Raut, A. V. 2017. Socio-demographic determinants of out-of-pocket health expenditure in a rural area of Wardha district of Maharashtra, India. *The Indian Jjournal of Medical Research* 146(5): 654.

Lohrisch, C., Paltiel, C., Gelmon, K., Speers, C., Taylor, S., Barnett, J., & Olivotto, I. A. (2006). Impact on survival of time from definitive surgery to initiation of adjuvant chemotherapy for early-stage breast cancer. *Journal of Clinical Oncology* 24(30):4888-4894.

Longo, C. J., & Bereza, B. G. 2011. A comparative analysis of monthly out-of-pocket costs for patients with breast cancer as compared with other common cancers in Ontario, Canada. *Current Oncology* 18(1):e1

Lwanga, S. K., Lemeshow, S., & World Health Organization. 1991. Sample size determination in health studies: a practical manual.

Malaysian Medical Council. 2013. Annual Reports. Kuala Lumpur. Malaysian Medical Council. http://mmc.gov.my/v1/index.php?option=com_content&task=view&id=86&Itemid=129

Malaysian National Cancer Registry Report 2007-11

Malin, J. L., Schneider, E. C., Epstein, A. M., Adams, J., Emanuel, E. J., & Kahn, K. L. 2006. Results of the National Initiative for Cancer Care Quality: how can we improve the quality of cancer care in the United States. *J Clin Oncol* 24(4): 626-634.

Marshall, M. N., Shekelle, P. G., McGlynn, E. A., Campbell, S., Brook, R. H., & Roland, M. O. 2003. Can health care quality indicators be transferred between countries? *BMJ Quality & Safety* 12(1):8-12.

Mathauer, I., Xu, K., Carrin, G., & Evans, D. B. 2009. *An Analysis of the Health Financing System of the Republic of Korea and Options to Strengthen Health Financing Performance.* World Health Organization. Geneva: Swiss 29-30.

Matsaganis, M., Mitrakos, T., & Tsakloglou, P. 2009. Modelling health expenditure at the household level in Greece. *The European Journal of Health Economics* 10(3):329-336.

Maunsell, E., Drolet, M., Brisson, J., Brisson, C., Mâsse, B., & Deschênes, L. 2004. Work situation after breast cancer: results from a population-based study. *Journal of the National Cancer Institute* 96(24):1813-1822.

Mcintyre, D., Meheus, F., & Røttingen, J. A. 2017. What level of domestic government health expenditure should we aspire to for universal health coverage? *Health Economics, Policy and Law* 12(2): 125-137.

McLaughlin, J. M., Anderson, R. T., Ferketich, A. K., Seiber, E. E., Balkrishnan, R., & Paskett, E. D. 2012. Effect on survival of longer intervals between confirmed diagnosis and treatment initiation among low-income women with breast cancer. *Journal of Clinical Oncology* 30(36):4493.

Mechili, A., Zimeras, S., Al-Fantel, K., & Diomidous, M. 2014. The use of geographical information system in health sector. In *ICIMTH*:185-188).

Mejin, M., Keowmani, T., Rahman, S. A., Liew, J., Lai, J., Chua, M., & Wan, I. C. 2019. Prevalence of pain and treatment outcomes among cancer patients in a Malaysian palliative care unit. *Pharmacy practice*, *17*(1)

Micklewright, J., & Schnepf, S. V. 2010. How reliable are income data collected with a single question? *Journal of the Royal Statistical Society: Series A (Statistics in Society)* 173(2):409-429.

Ministry of Education. 2014. Hala Tuju Pendidikan Farmasi (2011-2015). https://www.moe.gov.my/index.php/en/media/penerbitan/terbitan/rujukan-akademik/1397-hala-tuju-pendidikan-farmasi-2011-2015.

MOH. 2010a. Clinical practice guidelines on the management of breast cancer. 2nd Edition. MOH/P/PAK.212.10(GU).

MOH. 2010b. Clinical practice guidelines on the management of cancer pain. MOH/P/PAK/205.10(GU).

MOH. 2010c. Palliative care services operational policy. MOH/P/PAK/203.10(BP).

MOH. 2011. *Garispanduan Program Pengesanan Awal Kanser Payu Dara.*

MOH. 2012. *Malaysian National Medicines Policy.* 2nd edition. https://www.pharmacy.gov.my/v2/ [11 July 2015].

MOH. 2015a. *Human resources for health country profiles 2015 Malaysia.*

MOH. 2015b. Director General of Health keynote address: managing breast cancer in Malaysia, at the 13th Asian Breast Disease Association (ABDA) teaching course. https://kpkesihatan.com/2015/08/03/dg-of-healths-keynote-address-vision-of-the-future-managing-breast-cancer-in-malaysia-at-the-13th-asian-breast-diseases-association-abda-teaching-course/

MOH. 2016a. *The National Strategic Plan for Cancer Control Programme (NSPCCP) 2016-2020.*

MOH. 2016b. *Systemic Therapy Protocol.* 3rd edition. MOH/P/IKN/02.17(BK).

MOH. 2016c. *Malaysia National Health Accounts Health Expenditure Report 1997-2015.*

MOH. 2016d. *National Essential Medicines List.* 4th Edition. https://www.pharmacy.gov.my/v2/sites/default/files/document-upload/national-essential-medicines-list-fourth-edition.pdf. [11 July 2017].

MOH 2016e. *Health Facts 2015.* vlib.moh.gov.my/cms/content. [15 May 2016].

Mohamad Shofi Mat Isa. 2016. Tanda kasih suami sanggup berhenti kerja. Utusan Online, 23 June, http://www.utusan.com.my/berita/nasional/tanda-kasih-suami-sanggup-berhenti-kerja-1.345947. [7 July 2016].

Mohamed Sahidi Yusof. 2016. POKB bantu pesakit kanser tahap tiga. BH Online, 23 October. https://www.bharian.com.my/node/205095. [7 July 2016].

Mohammed J, Ashton T, North N. Wave upon wave: Fiji's experiments in decentralizing its health care system. Asia Pac J Public Health. 2016;28(3):232–243.

Moore, J. C., & Welniak, E. J. 2000. Income measurement error in surveys: A review. *Journal of Official Statistics* 16(4):331.

Moradi, G., Safari, H., Piroozi, B., Qanbari, L., Farshadi, S., Qasri, H., & Farhadifar, F. 2017. Catastrophic health expenditure among households with members with special diseases: A case study in Kurdistan. *Medical journal of the Islamic Republic of Iran* 31:43.

Musa, G.J., Chiang, P.H., Sylk, T., Bavley, R., Keating, W., Lakew, B., Tsou, H.C. and Hoven, C.W. 2013. Use of GIS Mapping as a Public Health Tool—From Cholera to Cancer. *Health services insights* 6:S10471.

Mwai, D., & Muriithi, M. 2016. Catastrophic Health Expenditure and Household Impoverishment: a case of NCDs prevalence in Kenya. *Epidemiology, Biostatistics and Public Health* 13(1).

National Collaborating Centre for Cancer UK. 2009. Early and locally advanced breast cancer: diagnosis and treatment. https://www.nice.org.uk/ (15 July 2015). [1 July 2015].

National Economic Advisory Council, 2010. *New economic model for Malaysia Part I: Strategic Policy Directions, Malaysia Document.*

Ng, M., Fullman, N., Dieleman, J. L., Flaxman, A. D., Murray, C. J., & Lim, S. S. 2014. Effective coverage: a metric for monitoring universal health coverage. *PLoS Medicine* 11(9): e1001730.

Ng, C. 2015. *Universal Health Coverage Assesssment: Malaysia.* Global Network for Health Equity (GNHE).

National Institute for Health and Care Excellence (NICE). n.d. Breast cancer quality standard. https://www.nice.org.uk/guidance/qs12/resources/breast-cancer-pdf. [1 July 2015].

O'Donnell, O., Van Doorslaer, E., Wagstaff, A., & Lindelow, M. 2007. *Analyzing health equity using household survey data: a guide to techniques and their implementation.* The World Bank.

OECD/WHO. 2016. Health at a Glance: Asia/Pacific 2016: Measuring Progress towards Universal Health Coverage, OECD Publishing, Paris, https://doi.org/10.1787/health_glance_ap-2016-en.[5 August 2017].

OECD. 2017. *Population Coverage for Health Care in Health at a Glance 2017:* OECD Indicators, OECD Publishing, Paris.

Parkin, D. M., Bray, F., Ferlay, J., & Pisani, P. 2005. Global cancer statistics, 2002. *CA: a cancer journal for clinicians*, 55(2), 74-108.

Pathy, N.B., Yip, C.H., Taib, N.A., Hartman, M., Saxena, N., Iau, P., Bulgiba, A.M., Lee, S.C., Lim, S.E., Wong, J.E. and Verkooijen, H.M. 2011. Breast cancer in a multi-ethnic Asian setting: results from the Singapore–Malaysia hospital-based breast cancer registry. *The Breast* 20:S75-S80.

Piccart-Gebhart, M.J., Procter, M., Leyland-Jones, B., Goldhirsch, A., Untch, M., Smith, I., Gianni, L., Baselga, J., Bell, R., Jackisch, C. and Cameron, D. 2005. Trastuzumab after adjuvant chemotherapy in HER2-positive breast cancer. *New England Journal of Medicine* 353(16):1659-1672.

Rajpal, S., Kumar, A., & Joe, W. 2018. Economic burden of cancer in India: Evidence from cross-sectional nationally representative household survey, 2014. *PloS One* 13(2):e0193320.

Recht, Abram, Elizabeth A. Comen, Richard E. Fine, Gini F. Fleming, Patricia H. Hardenbergh, Alice Y. Ho, Clifford A. Hudis et al. 2016. Postmastectomy radiotherapy: n American society of clinical oncology, American society for radiation oncology, and society of surgical oncology focused guideline update. *Practical Radiation Oncology* 6(6):e219-e234.

Redda, M. R., Verna, R., Guarneri, A., & Sannazzari, G. L. 2002. Timing of radiotherapy in breast cancer conserving treatment. *Cancer Treatment Reviews* 28(1):5-10.

Roberts, R. O., Bergstralh, E. J., Schmidt, L., & Jacobsen, S. J. 1996. Comparison of self-reported and medical record health care utilization measures. *Journal of Clinical Epidemiology* 49(9):989-995.

Robertson, J., Barr, R., Shulman, L. N., Forte, G. B., & Magrini, N. 2016. Essential medicines for cancer: WHO recommendations and national priorities. *Bulletin of the World Health Organization* 94(10):735.

Rockefeller Foundation Center, Bellagio. 2012. Measurement of trends and equity in coverage of health interventions in the context of universal health coverage. https://www.who.int/healthinfo/country_monitoring_evaluation/UHC_MeetinM_Bellagio_Sep2012_Report.pdf. [1 July 2015].

Romond, E.H., Perez, E.A., Bryant, J., Suman, V.J., Geyer Jr, C.E., Davidson, N.E., Tan-Chiu, E., Martino, S., Paik, S., Kaufman, P.A. and Swain, S.M. 2005. Trastuzumab plus adjuvant chemotherapy for operable HER2-positive breast cancer. *New England Journal of Medicine* 353(16):1673-1684.

Ruger, J. P., & Kim, H. J. 2007. Out-of-pocket healthcare spending by the poor and chronically ill in the Republic of Korea. *American Journal of Public Health* 97(5): 804-811.

Ruiterkamp, J., Ernst, M. F., Van de Poll-Franse, L. V., Bosscha, K., Tjan-Heijnen, V. C. G., & Voogd, A. C. 2009. Surgical resection of the primary tumour is associated with improved survival in patients with distant metastatic breast cancer at diagnosis. *European Journal of Surgical Oncology* 35(11):1146-1151.

Saito, N., Takahashi, M., Sairenchi, T., & Muto, T. 2014. The impact of breast cancer on employment among Japanese women. *Journal of occupational health*, 13-0140.

Sankaranarayanan, R., Swaminathan, R., Jayant, K., & Brenner, H. 2011. An overview of cancer survival in Africa, Asia, the Caribbean and Central America: the case for investment in cancer health services. *IARC Sci Publ* 162: 257-291.

Savedoff, W. 2005. How much should countries spend on health? *Health for the Millions* 5-10.

Savedoff, W. D. 2007. What should a country spend on health care? *Health Affairs* 26(4): 962-970.

Savedoff, W. D., de Ferranti, D., Smith, A. L., & Fan, V. 2012. Political and economic aspects of the transition to universal health coverage. *The Lancet* 380(9845):924-932.

Savedoff, W. D., & Smith, A. L. 2011. Achieving universal health coverage: learning from Chile, Japan, Malaysia and Sweden. *Washington, DC: Results for Development Institute.*

Senkus, E., Kyriakides, S., Penault-Llorca, F., Poortmans, P., Thompson, A., Zackrisson, S., Cardoso, F. and ESMO Guidelines Working Group. 2013. Primary breast cancer: ESMO Clinical Practice Guidelines for diagnosis, treatment and follow-up. *Annals of Oncology* 24(6):vi7-vi23.

Seya, M. J., Gelders, S. F., Achara, O. U., Milani, B., & Scholten, W. K. (2011). A first comparison between the consumption of and the need for opioid analgesics at country, regional, and global levels. *Journal of pain & palliative care pharmacotherapy*, 25(1), 6-18.

Shen, Y. C., & McFeeters, J. 2006. Out-of-pocket health spending between low-and higher-income populations: who is at risk of having high expenses and high burdens? *Medical Care* 200-209.

Shukla, M., Monika Agarwal, M., Singh, J., Tripathi, A., Srivastava, A., & Singh, V. K. 2015. Catastrophic health ex-penditure amongst people living with HIV/AIDS availing antiretro-viral treatment services at two tertiary care health facilities in district of Northern India. *Ntl J of Community Med* 6(3):323-8.

Shulman, L. N., Torode, J., Wagner, C., de Lima Lopes Jr, G., Barr, R., & Magrini, N. 2016. WHO expands cancer essential medicines list. Available at: am. asco. org/daily-news/who-expands-cancer-essential-medicines-list. [3 July 2016].

Sivalal S. Health technology assessment in the Asia Pacific region. Int J Technol Assess Health Care. 2009;25(Suppl 1):196–201.

Slamon, D., Eiermann, W., Robert, N., Pienkowski, T., Martin, M., Press, M., Mackey, J., Glaspy, J., Chan, A., Pawlicki, M. and Pinter, T. 2011. Adjuvant trastuzumab in HER2-positive breast cancer. *New England Journal of Medicine* 365(14):1273-1283.

Somkotra, T., & Lagrada, L. P. 2009. Which households are at risk of catastrophic health spending: experience in Thailand after universal coverage. *Health Affairs* 28(3): w467-w478.

Souza, C. B., Fustinoni, S. M., Amorim, M. H. C., Zandonade, E., Matos, J. C., & Schirmer, J. 2015. Breast cancer: diagnosis-to-treatment waiting times for elderly women at a reference hospital of São Paulo, Brazil. *Ciencia & saude coletiva* 20(12):3805-3816.

Stuckler, D., Feigl, A. B., Basu, S., & McKee, M. 2010. The political economy of universal health coverage. Background paper for the global symposium on health systems research.

Organisation for Economic Co-operation and Development.1991. *OECD Health Data: A Comparative Analysis of 30 Countries.* OECD.

Ramachandran, R., & Jha, V. 2013. Kidney transplantation is associated with catastrophic out of pocket expenditure in India. *PLoS One* 8(7):e67812.

Rasanathan K, Posayanonda T, Birmingham M, Tangcharoensathien V. Innovation and participation for healthy public policy: the First National Health Assembly in Thailand. Health Expect. 2012;15(1):87–96.

Tangcharoensathien, V., Patcharanarumol, W., Ir, P., Aljunid, S. M., Mukti, A. G., Akkhavong, K., ... & Mills, A. (2011). Health-financing reforms in southeast Asia: challenges in achieving universal coverage. *The Lancet, 377*(9768), 863-873.)

The World Bank. 2013. Out-Of-Pocket Health Expenditure (% Of Total Expenditure On Health). https://datacatalog.worldbank.org/out-pocket-health-expenditure-total-expenditure-health. [1 July 2015].

The World Bank. 2015. Why did the World Bank decide to update the International Poverty Line? https://datahelpdesk.worldbank.org/knowledgebase/articles. [10 May 2017].

Thomas, J.M., Fitzharris, B.M., Redding, W.H., Williams, J.E., Trott, P.A., Powles, T.J., Ford, H.T. and Gazet, J.C. 1978. Clinical examination, xeromammography, and fine-needle aspiration cytology in diagnosis of breast tumours. *BMJ* 2(6145):1139-1141.

Timmons, A., Sharp, L., Carsin, A.E., Donnelly, N., Kelly, J., McCormack, J., Chonghaile, N., O'Donnell, E., Ryan, O. and Comber, H. 2009. The cost of having cancer: a survey of patients with cancer in Ireland. *Journal of Epidemiology & Community Health* 63(2):46-46.

Toi, M., Ohashi, Y., Seow, A., Moriya, T., Tse, G., Sasano, H., Park, B.W., Chow, L.W., Laudico, A.V., Yip, C.H. and Ueno, E. 2010. The Breast Cancer Working Group presentation was divided into three sections: the epidemiology, pathology and treatment of breast cancer. *Japanese Journal of Clinical Oncology* 40(1): i13-i18.

Turrell, G. 2000. Income non-reporting: implications for health inequalities research. *Journal of Epidemiology & Community Health* 54(3):207-214.

Unit, E. I. 2015. The 2015 quality of death index. Ranking palliative care across the world. 2015. *The Economist Group*, London.

United Nations. (n.d.). About the sustainable development goals. https://www.un.org/sustainabledevelopment/sustainable-development-goals/[5 July 2015].

United Nations 2012 - Political declaration of the High-level Meeting of the General Assembly on the Prevention and Control of Non-communicable Diseases. In: General Assembly of the United Nations. Sixty-sixth session of the General Assembly of the United Nations, New York, 19–20 September 2012. New York: United Nations; 2012 (A/RES/66/2).

United Nations Development Group. 2003. Indicators for monitoring the Millennium Development Goals. New York, United Nations, 2003 (http://devdata.worldbank.org/gmis/mdg/UNDG%20document_final.pdf/[5 July 2015].

USAID/Health Systems 20/20. 2012. *Measuring and Monitoring Country Progress Towards Universal Health Coverage: Concepts, Indicators, and Experiences.* Meeting Summary. 20 July. Washington DC.

Van Doorslaer, E., O'Donnell, O., Rannan-Eliya, R.P., Somanathan, A., Adhikari, S.R., Garg, C.C., Harbianto, D., Herrin, A.N., Huq, M.N., Ibragimova, S. and Karan, A. 2006. Effect of payments for health care on poverty estimates in 11 countries in Asia: an analysis of household survey data. *The Lancet* 368(9544):1357-1364.

Van Minh, H., Phuong, N. T. K., Saksena, P., James, C. D., & Xu, K. 2013. Financial burden of household out-of pocket health expenditure in Viet Nam: findings from the National Living Standard Survey 2002–2010. *Social Science & Medicine* 96:258-263.

Van Minh, H., & Xuan Tran, B. 2012. Assessing the household financial burden associated with the chronic non-communicable diseases in a rural district of Vietnam. *Global Health Action* 5(1):18892.

Wagstaff, A., & Doorslaer, E. V. 2003. Catastrophe and impoverishment in paying for health care: with applications to Vietnam 1993–1998. *Health Economics* 12(11): 921-933.

Wagstaff, A., Cotlear, D., Eozenou, P. H. V., & Buisman, L. R. 2016. Measuring progress towards universal health coverage: with an application to 24 developing countries. *Oxford Review of Economic Policy* 32(1): 147-189.

Walter, L. C., Davidowitz, N. P., Heineken, P. A., & Covinsky, K. E. 2004. Pitfalls of converting practice guidelines into quality measures: lessons learned from a VA performance measure. *JAMA* 291(20):2466-2470.

Weedon-Fekjær, H., Romundstad, P. R., & Vatten, L. J. 2014. Modern mammography screening and breast cancer mortality: population study. *BMJ* 348: g3701.

WHO Global Health Expenditure Database. http://apps.who.int/nha/database. [1 July 2015].

WHO. n.d. WHO Definition of Palliative Care https://www.who.int/cancer/palliative/definition/en/. [1 May 2016].

WHO. 1981. Global strategy for health for all by the year 2000 (No. 3). World Health Organization.

WHO. 2003. *How Much Should Countries Spend on Health?* Geneva, Switzerland: World Health Organization.

WHO. 2006. *Working together for Health: The World Health Report 2006.*

WHO. 2008. *Health Metrics Network.* Geneva: WHO. http://www.who.int/healthmetrics/about/history/en (7 July 2015).

WHO. 2010a. *World Health Report, 2010: Health Systems Financing the Path to Universal Coverage.*

WHO. 2010b. *Monitoring the Building Blocks of Health Systems: A Handbook of Indicators and Their Measurement Strategies.* World Health Organization.

WHO. 2011. Validity and comparability of out-of-pocket health expenditure from household surveys: a review of the literature and current survey instruments.

WHO. 2013a. *Draft Comprehensive Global Monitoring Framework and Targets for the Prevention and Control of Non-communicable Diseases.* Geneva: World Health Organization, 15.

WHO. 2013b. *Global Action Plan for the Prevention and Control of NCDs 2013-2020.* Geneva: World Health Organization.

WHO. 2013c. Service Availability and Readiness Assessment (SARA): An Annual Monitoring System for Service Delivery. Reference manual.

WHO. 2013d. WHO Model List of Essential Medicines. http://www.who.int/medicines/publications/essentialmedicines/en/index.html

WHO. 2014a. Monitoring Progress towards Universal Health Coverage at Country and Global Levels: Framework, Measures and Targets. WHO/HIS/HIA/14.1. World Health Organization.

WHO. 2014b. Human resources country profiles: Malaysia.

WHO. 2015. Tracking Universal Health Coverage: First Global Monitoring Report. World Health Organization.

WHO. 2016a. Universal health coverage: moving towards better health: action framework for the Western Pacific Region.

WHO. 2016b. Health workforce requirements for universal health coverage and the Sustainable Development Goals. Human Resources for Health Observer, 17.

World Health Organization (WHO) Regional Office for the Western Pacific. Universal health coverage: moving towards better health: action framework for the Western Pacific Region. Manila (Philippines): WHO Regional Office for the WesternPacific; 2016.http://www.who.int/iris/handle/10665/246420. [2 November 2017]

WHO. 2017. *Out-of-pocket Payments, User Fees and Catastrophic* Expenditure. World Health Organization.

Wolff, E. N. 1998. Recent trends in the size distribution of household wealth. Journal of Economic Perspectives 12(3):131-150.

World Health Assembly. 2013. Resolution EB 132/7. Draft action plan for the prevention and control of noncommunicable diseases 2013–2020. Geneva: World Health Assembly

Worldwide Hospice Palliative Care Alliance. 2014. Universal Health Coverage and Palliative Care. http://www.thewhpca.org/images/resources/publications-reports/Universal_health_coverage_report_final_2014.pdf [1 July 2015].

Xu, K., Evans, D. B., Kawabata, K., Zeramdini, R., Klavus, J., & Murray, C. J. 2003. Household catastrophic health expenditure: a multicountry analysis. The Lancet 362(9378):111-117.

Xu, K., & World Health Organization. 2005. Distribution of Health Payments and Catastrophic Expenditures Methodology (No. EIP/FER/DP. 05.2). Geneva: World Health Organization.

Xu, K., Evans, D. B., Carrin, G., Aguilar-Rivera, A. M., Musgrove, P., & Evans, T. (2007). Protecting households from catastrophic health spending. *Health Affairs* 26(4):972-983.

Yang, T., Chu, J., Zhou, C., Medina, A., Li, C., Jiang, S., Zheng, W., Sun, L. and Liu, J. 2016. Catastrophic health expenditure: a comparative analysis of empty-nest and non-empty-nest households with seniors in Shandong, China. *BMJ Open* 6(7):e010992.

Yardim, M. S., Cilingiroglu, N., & Yardim, N. 2010. Catastrophic health expenditure and impoverishment in Turkey. *Health Policy* 94(1):26-33.

Yeong-Sheng, T. E. Y. 2008. *Household expenditure on food at home in Malaysia*. University Library of Munich, Germany.

Yip, C.H., Smith, R.A., Anderson, B.O., Miller, A.B., Thomas, D.B., Ang, E.S., Caffarella, R.S., Corbex, M., Kreps, G.L., McTiernan, A. and Breast Health Global Initiative Early Detection Panel. 2008. Guideline implementation for breast healthcare in low-and middle-income countries: early detection resource allocation. *Cancer* 113(S8):2244-2256.

Youlden, D. R., Cramb, S. M., Yip, C. H., & Baade, P. D. 2014. Incidence and mortality of female breast cancer in the Asia-Pacific region. *Cancer Biology & Medicine* 11(2):101.

Yu, K. D., Huang, S., Zhang, J. X., Liu, G. Y., & Shao, Z. M. 2013. Association between delayed initiation of adjuvant CMF or anthracycline-based chemotherapy and survival in breast cancer: a systematic review and meta-analysis. *BMC Cancer* 13(1):240.

Zaidi, S., Bigdeli, M., Aleem, N., & Rashidian, A. 2013. Access to essential medicines in Pakistan: policy and health systems research concerns. *PloS One* 8(5):e63515.

Ziller, E. C., Coburn, A. F., & Yousefian, A. E. 2006. Out-of-pocket health spending and the rural underinsured. *Health Affairs* 25(6): 1688-1699.

Zulkipli, A.F., Islam, T., Mohd Taib, N.A., Dahlui, M., Bhoo-Pathy, N., Al-Sadat, N., Abdul Majid, H. and Hussain, S. 2018. Use of Complementary and Alternative Medicine Among Newly Diagnosed Breast Cancer Patients in Malaysia: An Early Report From the MyBCC Study. *Integrative cancer therapies* 17(2):312-321.

Zuma, S. M. 2013. The factors affecting availability of medicines in the Free State District Health Services. Doctoral dissertation.

Appendix A1

INDICATORS FOR UHC MONITORING (USAID JULY 2012)

Indicator	Source
Service utilization (Percentage of relevant populations)	
Births delivered in a health facility	DHS
Births assisted by a skilled provider	DHS; UNICEF/UNFPA; WHO database
Women receiving ANC from a skilled provider	DHS; UN MDGs Indicators; WHO, UNICEF
Married women in reproductive age using modern FP method	DHS; World Contraceptive Use 2011 (UN, 2011)
Family Planning Needs Satisfied	DHS
Received all basic vaccines	DHS; WHO database
Received Measles vaccine	DHS; WHO database
Received 3 doses of DPT vaccine	DHS; WHO database
Received BCG vaccine	DHS; WHO database
Received ORT and continued feeding for diarrhoea treatment	DHS; MICS; UNICEF
Sought Treatment for ARI	DHS; MICS
Children under 5 with fever who received anti-malarial drugs	DHS; WHO database

Population with advanced HIV and access to ART drugs	UN MDGs Indicators
Other service/tracer indicators	
Households with at least one mosquito net	DHS for select countries
Children under 5 sleeping under ITNs	DHS; WHO database; for select countries
Pregnant women sleeping under ITNs	DHS for select countries
TB treatment success rate under DOTS, percentage	UN MDGs Indicators
% of women with serious problems accessing health care	DHS for select countries
Service availability and service readiness	
Hospital beds per 10,000 population	WHO database, national HMIS
Providers (by type) per 10,000 population	WHO database
Health Centres per 100,000 population	WHO database
Median or average availability of 14 selected generic medicines (%)	WHO & HAI
Median consumer price ratio of 14 selected generic medicines	WHO & HAI
Service Readiness Index	Service Availability and Readiness Assessment
Service quality	
TBD (to be determined)	
Population Coverage	
Indicators above by subgroups (e.g. geographical, income groups) whenever possible	Household surveys with either household asset variables or expenditure data (e.g. DHS, expenditure surveys)

Appendix A2

INDICATORS FOR SERVICE COVERAGE (USAID SEPTEMBER 2012)

Indicator	Definition	Source
Service utilization indicators		
Births delivered in a health facility	Percentage of live births in the previous five years delivered in a health facility	DHS
Births assisted by a skilled provider	Percentage of live births in the previous five years attended by a skilled health provider	DHS; UNICEF/UNFPA; WHO Global Health Observatory database
Women receiving any antenatal care (ANC) from a skilled provider	Percentage of women age 15-49 who gave birth in the previous five years who received ANC at least once from a skilled health provider	DHS; UN MDGs Indicators; WHO Global Health Observatory database, UNICEF
Married women in reproductive age using modern family planning (FP) method	Percentage of women aged 15–49 years currently married or in union who are using (or whose partner is using) a modern contraceptive method	DHS

Family planning needs satisfied	Percentage of currently married women who say that they do not want any more children or that they want to wait 2 or more years before having another child, and are using contraception	DHS
Received all basic vaccines	Percentage of children aged 12–23 months who received a BCG vaccine, a measles vaccine and three doses each of DPT and polio vaccine excluding polio vaccine given at birth.	DHS; WHO Global Health Observatory database
Received measles vaccine	Percentage of children aged 12–23 months who are immunised against measles	DHS; WHO Global Health Observatory database, UNICEF
Received 3 doses of DPT vaccine	Percentage of children aged 12–23 months who received three doses of diphtheria, pertussis, and tetanus vaccine	DHS; WHO Global Health Observatory database; UNICEF
Received BCG vaccine	Percentage of children aged 12–23 months currently vaccinated against BCG	DHS; WHO Global Health Observatory database
Received oral rehydration therapy (ORT) and continued feeding for diarrhoea treatment	Percentage of children under-5 with diarrhoea in the past 2 weeks who received ORT (packets of oral rehydration salts, or recommended home fluids such as sugar salt-water solution) and continued feeding	DHS for select countries MICS; UNICEF

Sought treatment for acute respiratory infection (ARI)	Percentage of children aged 0–59 months who showed symptoms of ARI in the two weeks preceding the survey who sought care from a health provider	DHS; MICS
Received anti-malarial drugs	Percentage of children aged 0–59 months who had fever in the two weeks preceding the survey who received anti-malarial drugs	DHS for select countries; WHO Global Health Observatory database
Access to antiretroviral (ART) drugs	Percentage of population with advanced HIV infection with access to ART drugs	UN MDGs Indicators continue...

...continuation

Other service coverage tracer indicators

Households with at least one mosquito net	Percentage of households with at least one mosquito net (treated or untreated)	DHS for select countries
Children under 5 sleeping under insecticide-treated net (ITNs)	Percentage of children under five years of age who slept under an ITN the night before the survey	DHS for select countries; WHO Global Health Observatory database
Pregnant women sleeping under ITNs	Percentage of pregnant women age 15-49 who slept under an ITN the night before the survey	DHS for select countries
TB treatment success rate under directly observed treatment short course (DOTS)	Percentage of tuberculosis cases detected and cured under DOTS	UN MDGs Indicators

Percentage of women with serious problems in accessing health care	Percentage of women age 15-49 who reported that they have serious problems in accessing health care for themselves when they are sick	DHS for select countries

Appendix A3

INDICATORS FOR SERVICE COVERAGE (WHO & WBG 2014)

Area	Promotion and prevention	Treatment, Rehabilitation, Palliation
Pregnancy care	ANC (4+ visits); TT vaccination	Treatment of pregnant women with positive syphilis test
Maternal/ newborn care	Postnatal care for mother and newborn	Institutional delivery/ skilled birth attendance
Family planning	Need for family planning satisfied	
Child vaccination	DPT3/pentavalent, PCV, measles, BCG immunization; fully vaccinated	
Treatment of child illness		Pneumonia to health facility/received antibiotics; diarrhea with ORT/ORS
Child undernutrition	Exclusive breastfeeding; vitamin A supplementation; households with iodized salt	
Malaria control	ITN use among children/ pregnant women, household ownership, indoor residual spraying	Child with fever taken to facility/confirmed cases treated with first line antimalarial

TB Control		TB case detection rate, treatment success rate; HIV-TB patients receiving CPT
HIV prevention and treatment/STI	PMTCT among HIV positive women; voluntary HIV testing and counseling (general, risk populations); condom use at higher risk sex (general, risk populations)	Antiretroviral therapy; HIV and TB treatment among HIV infected persons with incident TB infection; STI appropriately diagnosed and treatment
Neglected tropical diseases (NTD)	Preventive treatment coverage among those at risk of NTD	Treatment among those with NTD
Epidemic prone diseases	Meningitis vaccination coverage; influenza vaccination	Treatment among those with epidemic disease
NCD	Non-use tobacco; adequate physical activity; non-obesity/overweight; non-heavy episodic use of alcohol; normal cholesterol	Hypertension treatment, diabetes treatment; preventive treatment among persons with elevated risk of severe cardiovascular events; CVD and stroke treatment; cardiac surgical interventions; cataract surgery
Cancer screening and vaccination	HPV vaccination; cervical cancer screening; mammography	Cancer treatment
Mental health		Depression treatment; severe mental disorder treatment
Surgical conditions		Hip/knee replacement, hernia, other types of surgery

Continue…

…continuation

Environmental health	Water supply from safe source; adequate sanitation	
	Exposure to good air quality	
	Modern fuels for indoor use	

	Helmet use; seatbelt use	
Injuries		Severe injury treatment
Rehabilitation		Assistive devices among persons with disabilities; rehabilitative surgical interventions; corrected refractive errors
Palliation		Use of opiates among those in need

Appendix A4

INDICATORS FOR UHC MONITORING (WHO & WBG 2015)

Indicator	Primary data source	Numerator	Denominator	Equity measurement available for this report
Promotion/prevention				
Family planning coverage with modern methods	Household surveys	Sexually active women 15–49 years who are currently using a modern contraceptive method	Women 15–49 years of age who are sexually active and do not wish to become pregnant	Wealth, education, urban/rural residence
Antenatal care coverage	Household surveys, administrative records	At least 4 visits to any care provider during pregnancy	Live births	Wealth, education, urban/rural residence

253

Skilled birth attendance	Household surveys, administrative records	Live births attended by skilled health personnel (doctors, nurses or midwives)	Live births	Wealth, education, urban/rural residence
Diphtheria, tetanus and pertussis (DTP3) immunization coverage among 1-year-olds	Administrative records	1-year-old children who have received 3 doses of a vaccine containing diphtheria, tetanus and pertussis	1-year-old children	Wealth, education, urban/rural residence, sex
Prevalence of no tobacco smoking in the past 30 days among adults age ≥ 15 years	Household surveys	Adults 15 years and older who have not smoked tobacco in the past 30 days	Adults 15 years and older	Sex
Percentage of population using improved drinking water sources	Household surveys	Population living in a household with drinking water from: piped water into dwelling, plot or yard; public tap/ stand pipe; tube well/ borehole; protected dug well; protected spring; or rainwater collection	Total population	Wealth, urban/rural Residence

Continue…

...continuation

Percentage of population using improved sanitation facilities	Household surveys	Population living in a household with: flush or pour-flush to piped sewer system, septic tank or pit latrine; ventilated improved pit latrine; pit latrine with slab; or composting toilet	Total population	Wealth, urban/rural residence
Preventive chemotherapy (PC) coverage against neglected tropical diseases (NTDs)	Administrative records	People requiring PC who have received PC (at least one NTD)	People requiring PC (at least one NTD)	None
Treatment indicators				
Antiretroviral therapy coverage	Administrative records, household surveys including HIV test	People who are currently receiving antiretroviral combination therapy	People living with HIV	None
Tuberculosis treatment coverage	Administrative records	New cases of TB that have been diagnosed and completed treatment each year	New cases of TB in a given year	None

Hypertension coverage	Health examination surveys including blood pressure measurement	Adults 18 years and older currently taking antihypertensive medication	Adults 18 years and older taking medication for hypertension, with systolic blood pressure ≥ 140 mmHg, or with diastolic blood pressure ≥ 90 mmHg	Wealth, sex
Diabetes coverage	Health examination surveys including blood glucose measurement	Adults 18 years and older currently taking medication for diabetes (insulin or glycaemic control pills)	Adults 18 years and older taking medication for diabetes or with fasting plasma glucose ≥7.0 mmol/l	Sex

Continue.... |
| ...continuation Cataract surgical coverage | Health examination surveys including visual acuity and basic causes of vision impairment | Adults 50 years and older who have received bilateral cataract surgery or who have received unilateral cataract surgery with operable cataract and visual acuity < 6/18 in the unoperated eye | Adults 50 years and older with bilateral operable cataract and visual acuity < 6/18, who have received cataract surgery in both eyes, or who have received cataract surgery in one eye and have operable cataract with visual acuity < 6/18 in the unoperated eye | Sex |

Appendix A5

NICCQ INDICATORS

Breast cancer treatment	NICCQ indicators
Surgery	• IF a patient with stage I-III breast cancer undergoes mastectomy as first therapeutic procedure, THEN prior to undergoing mastectomy, the patient should be informed about the option to have either breast conserving surgery followed by radiation therapy or mastectomy.
	• IF a patient with stage I-III breast cancer undergoes mastectomy, THEN prior to undergoing mastectomy the patient should be informed about the option of breast reconstruction after mastectomy.
Chemotherapy	• IF a patient newly diagnosed with stage II-III breast cancer is 50 years old and the tumour is 2 cm or the tumour involves the lymph nodes and is treated with chemotherapy, THEN the patient should start adjuvant chemotherapy within 8 weeks of the last therapeutic surgery
	• IF a patient is treated with chemotherapy, THEN the planned dose (dose per cycle _ number of cycles) should be documented in the medical oncology or integrated record

	• IF a patient is treated with chemotherapy, THEN the planned dose (dose per cycle _ number of cycles) should fall within a range that is consistent with published regimens
	• IF a patient is treated with chemotherapy, THEN body surface area should be documented
Radiation therapy	• IF a patient with a diagnosis of stage I-III breast cancer is treated with radiation therapy, THEN the radiation therapy medical record should document all of the following: (1) The total radiation dose, (2) the radiation dose per fraction or number of fractions given, (3) the site.
	• IF a patient with invasive breast cancer who undergoes a mastectomy has any of the following: (1) Positive margins on the surgical specimen, OR (2) tumour size _ 5 cm, OR (3) 4 or more involved lymph nodes, OR (4) a T4 lesion, THEN the patient should receive radiotherapy.
	• IF a patient with stage I-III breast cancer undergoes BCS (ie, does not have a mastectomy) and did not receive radiation therapy, THEN the patient should have a consultation with a radiation oncologist.
	• IF a patient with invasive breast cancer: (A) Undergoes a mastectomy AND (B) Has any of the following: (1) Positive margins on the surgical specimen, OR (2) tumour size 5 cm, OR (3) 4 or more involved lymph nodes, OR (4) aT4 lesion, THEN the patient should have a consultation with a radiation oncologist
Hormone therapy	• IF a patient with stage I-III breast cancer who initiates treatment with tamoxifen does not have evidence of disease progression, THEN the patient should receive 5 years of tamoxifen.
Targeted therapy	• Not available
Palliative care	• Not Available

Appendix A6

NICE INDICATORS

Breast cancer treatment	Indicators
Surgery	Not available
Chemotherapy	Not available
Radiation therapy	Not available
Hormone therapy	Not available
Targeted therapy	Not available
Palliative care	People with locally advanced, metastatic or distant recurrent breast cancer are assigned a key worker [2011, updated 2016]
Others	People with suspected breast cancer referred to specialist services are offered the triple diagnostic assessment in a single hospital visit [new 2016]
	People with biopsy-proven invasive breast cancer or ductal carcinoma in situ (DCIS) are not offered a preoperative MRI scan unless there are specific clinical indications for its use [new 2016],

People with oestrogen receptor-positive (ER-positive), human epidermal growth factor receptor 2-negative (HER2-negative) and lymph node-negative early breast cancer who are at intermediate risk of distant recurrence are offered gene expression profiling with Oncotype DX [new 2016]

People with newly diagnosed invasive breast cancer and those with recurrent breast cancer (if clinically appropriate) have the oestrogen receptor (ER) and human epidermal growth factor receptor 2 (HER2) status of the tumour assessed [2011, updated 2016]

People with breast cancer who develop metastatic disease have their treatment and care managed by a multidisciplinary team [2011, updated 2016]

Appendix A7

EUSOMA INDICATORS

Breast cancer treatment	European Society of Breast Cancer Specialists (EUSOMA) indicators
Surgery	Not available
Chemotherapy	Proportion of patients with ER (T > 1 cm or Node positive) invasive carcinoma who received adjuvant chemotherapy
	Proportion of patients with inflammatory breast cancer (IBC) or locally advanced non-resectable ER- carcinoma who received neo-adjuvant chemotherapy
Radiation therapy	Proportion of patients with invasive breast cancer (M0) who received postoperative radiation therapy (RT) after surgical resection of the primary tumour and appropriate axillary staging/surgery in the framework of BCT
	Proportion of patients with involvement of axillary lymph nodes (pN2a) who received post-mastectomy radiation therapy to the chest wall and all (non-resected) regional lymph-nodes
	Proportion of patients with involvement of up to three axillary lymph nodes (pN1) who received post-mastectomy radiation therapy to the chest wall and non-resected axillary lymph-nodes, including level IV (supraclavicular), and in medially located tumours, the internal mammary lymph-nodes

Hormone therapy	Proportion of patients with endocrine sensitive invasive cancer who received endocrine therapy
Targeted therapy	Proportion of patients with HER2 positive (IHC 3þ or in situ hybridisation positive FISH-positive) invasive carcinoma (T > 1 cm or Nþ) treated with chemotherapy who received adjuvant trastuzumab
	Proportion of patients with HER2-positive invasive carcinoma treated with neoadjuvant chemotherapy who received neo-adjuvant trastuzumab
Palliative care	Not available

Appendix A8

INDICATORS FOR HEALTH SYSTEM GOVERNANCE

Number	Indicators
1	Existence of an up-to-date national health strategy linked to national needs and priorities.
2	Existence and year of last update of a published national medicines policy.
3	Existence of policies on medicines procurement that specify the most cost-effective medicines in the right quantities; open, competitive bidding of suppliers of quality products.
4	Tuberculosis—existence of a national strategic plan for tuberculosis that reflects the six principal components of the Stop-TB strategy as outlined in the Global Plan to Stop TB 2006–2015.
5	Malaria—existence of a national malaria strategy or policy that includes drug efficacy monitoring, vector control and insecticide resistance monitoring.
6	HIV/AIDS—completion of the UNGASS National Composite Policy Index data collection form for HIV/AIDS.
7	Maternal health—existence of a comprehensive reproductive health policy consistent with the ICPD action plan.
8	Child health—existence of an updated comprehensive, multiyear plan for childhood immunization.

9	Existence of key health sector documents that are disseminated regularly (such as budget documents, annual performance reviews and health indicators).
10	Existence of mechanisms, such as surveys, for obtaining opportune client input on appropriate, timely and effective access to health services.

Appendix A9

INDICATORS FOR HEALTH SYSTEMS FINANCING

Indicators	Definition	Source of data
Total expenditure on health (TEH)	sum of all outlays for health maintenance, restoration or enhancement paid for in cash or supplied in kind. It is the sum of General Government Expenditure on Health and Private Expenditure on Health (WHO).	National Health Accounts (NHA).
General government expenditure on health as a proportion of general government expenditure	defined as the level of general government expenditure on health (GGHE) expressed as a percentage of total government expenditure (WHO).	National Health Accounts (NHA).

TEH as a percentage of GDP	the level of total expenditure on health (THE) expressed as a percentage of gross domestic product (GDP) (WHO).	National Health Accounts (NHA).
Ratio of household out-of-pocket payments for health to total expenditure on health	the level of out-of-pocket expenditure expressed as a percentage of private expenditure on health.	Household expenditure and utilization survey

Appendix A10
INDICATORS FOR HISPIX

Indicators
Health surveys
Country has a 10-year costed survey plan that covers all priority health topics and considers other relevant data sources.
Census
Census completed within the past 10 years
Population projections for districts and smaller administrative areas available for next 10 years, in print and electronically, well documented.
Health facility reporting
Country web site for health statistics, with latest report and data available to the general public
Health system resource tracking
At least one national health accounts exercise completed in the past five years
National database with public and private sector health facilities and geocoding, available and updated within the past three years

National database with health workers by district and main cadres updated within the past two years

Annual data on availability of tracer medicines and commodities in public and private health facilities

A designated and functioning institutional mechanism charged with analysis of health statistics, synthesis of data from different sources and validation of data from population-based and facility-based sources

A burden of disease study conducted within the past five years, with a strong national contribution

A health systems performance assessment carried out within the past five years, with a strong national contribution

Appendix A11

INDICATORS FOR ESSENTIAL MEDICINES

Source	Indicators	Formula	Target
MDG Target 8E	Availability of 14 essential medicines	The number of facilities with all 14 essential medicines in stock (present and not expired) on the day of visit / Total number of facilities surveyed in sample area) x 100.	Not stated
WHO Handbook of Indicators and Measurements to monitor the building blocks of health system (2010)	Average availability of 14 essential medicines Median consumer price of 14 essential medicines.	As above The consumer price ratios for 14 essential medicines = ratio between median unit prices and the median international reference prices for that same product for the year preceding the survey	Not stated

WHO Global Action Plan for the Prevention and Control of NCDs 2013-2020 (2013).	Availability of the affordable basic technologies and essential medicines, including generics, required to treat major NCDs	Voluntary global target of 80% availability
WHO Essential Medicine List (EML) for cancer (2013 and 2016)	A useful framework for low- and middle-income countries (LMICs) to determine how best to invest resources in health care.	Voluntary global target of 80% availability

Appendix A12

MALAYSIAN NATIONAL ESSENTIAL MEDICINE LIST (2014) COMPARED TO THE WHO ESSENTIAL MEDICINES LIST (2013, 2015)

Drugs	Malaysian National Essential Medicine List (4th Ed)(2014)	WHO List of Essential Medicines (2013)	WHO List of Essential Medicines (2015)
OPIOID ANALGESICS			
Dihydrocodeine	Yes		
Morphine	Yes		
Tramadol	Yes		
Tramadol	Yes		
IMMUNOSUPPRESSIVE MEDICINES			
Azathioprine	Yes		
Cyclosporine	Yes		
Methotrexate	No	Yes	Yes

CYTOTOXIC & ADJUVANT MEDICINES

L-asparaginase	Yes	Yes	Yes
Bleomycin	Yes	Yes	Yes
Calcium folinate tab/inj	Yes	Yes	Yes
Carboplatin	Yes	Yes	Yes
Chlorambucil	Yes	Yes	Yes
Cyclophosphamide tab/inj	Yes	Yes	Yes
Cytarabine	Yes	Yes	Yes
Dacarbazine	Yes	Yes	Yes
Dactinomycin	Yes	Yes	Yes
Daunorubicin	Yes	Yes	Yes
Docetaxel	Yes	Yes	Yes
Doxorubicin	Yes	Yes	Yes
Etoposide tab/inj	Yes	Yes	Yes
Fluorouracil	Yes	Yes	Yes
Ifosfamide	Yes	Yes	Yes
Mercaptopurine	Yes	Yes	Yes
Paclitaxel	Yes	Yes	Yes
Procarbazine	Yes	Yes	Yes
Thioguanine	Yes	Yes	Yes
Vinblastine	Yes	Yes	Yes
Vincristine	Yes	Yes	Yes
ATRA	No		Yes
Bendamustine	No		Yes
Capecitabine	No		Yes
Cisplatin	No		Yes
Fludarabine	No		Yes
Gemcitabine	No		Yes

continue...

...continuation

Irinotecan	No		Yes
Oxaliplatin	No		Yes
Vinorelbine	No		Yes

HORMONES AND ANTIHORMONES

Tamoxifen	Yes	Yes	Yes
Anastrazole	No		Yes
Bicalutamide	No		Yes
Leuprolide	No		Yes

OTHERS

Allopurinol	No	Yes	Yes
Dexamethasone	No	Yes	Yes
Hydrocortisone	No	Yes	Yes
Hydroxyurea	No	Yes	Yes
Mesna	No	Yes	Yes
Methylprednisolone	No	Yes	Yes
Prednisolone	No	Yes	Yes
G-CSF	No		Yes
Imatinib	No		Yes
Rituximab	No		Yes
Trastuzumab	No		Yes

Appendix A13

SOURCES, INDICATORS AND TARGETS FOR HEALTH WORKFORCE

Source	Indicator	Formula	Target
World Health Report (2006)	Number of health workers per 10 000 population	Number of health workers (physicians and nurses/ midwives) per 10 000 population	Minimum health worker density of 2.3 skilled health workers per 1000 population
International Labour Organization ILO			3.4 skilled health workers per 1000 population.
WHO Handbook of Indicators and Measurements to monitor the building blocks of health system (2010)	Number of health workers per 10 000 population	The absolute number of health workers divided by the total population for the same geographical area.	

	Distribution of health workers~~by occupation~~/ specialization, region, place of work and sex	The number of health workers with a given characteristic divided by the total number of health workers.	
	Annual number of graduates of health professions educational institutions per 100 000 population – by level and field of education	The absolute number of graduates of health professions educational institutions in the past academic year (by level and field of education) divided by the total population	
Health Workforce Requirements for Universal Health Coverage and the Sustainable Development Goals Background Paper No. 1 to the Global Strategy on Human Resources for Health 2016).	The World Health Organization (WHO) Global Strategy on Human Resources for Health: Workforce 2030 sets out the policy agenda to ensure a workforce that is fit for purpose to attain the targets of the Sustainable Development Goals (SDGs)		4.45 skilled health workers per 1000 For doctors, the mean density in 2013 was 1.4 (SD 1.2) per 1000 population, while for nurses it was 4.1 (SD 2.8) per 1000 population.

Appendix A14

INDICATORS FOR HEALTH SERVICE DELIVERY

Source	Indicator	Formula	Notes
Handbook of Indicators and Measurements to monitor the building blocks of health system (WHO 2010)	**General service availability**		
	Number and distribution of health facilities per 10000 population	The number of health facilities divided by the total population for the same geographical area	Health facilities refer to all public and private health facilities, defined as a static facility (a designated building) in which general health services are offered. It does not include mobile service delivery points and non-formal services, such as traditional healers.

Number and distribution of inpatient beds per 10000 population	The number of inpatient beds divided by the total population for the same geographical area.	This includes total hospital beds (for long-term and acute care), maternity beds and paediatric beds, but not delivery beds. Public and private sectors are included.
Number of outpatient department visits per 10000 population per year	The number of visits to health facilities for ambulant care divided by the total population for the same geographical area.	Not including immunization (can be divided into children under five years of age and aged five years and over)

General service readiness

General service readiness for health facilities	Derived from data on availability and functioning of tracer items in the facility on the day of assessment	These items are grouped in five domains: basic amenities, basic equipment, and standard precautions for prevention of infections, laboratory, medicines and commodities.

Service-specific availability

Proportion of health facilities offering specific services

	Number and distribution of health facilities offering specific services per 10000 population	The number of facilities in which a specific service is offered divided by the total number of facilities (to obtain the proportion), or, the total population for the same geographical area (to compute the density)	
	Service-specific readiness		
	Service-specific readiness score for health facilities	Cumulative availability of components required in health facilities to deliver specific services, expressed as percentage.	Staff and training, equipment, diagnostics, medicines and commodities

Appendix B1

PATIENT INFORMATION SHEET
(BAHASA MALAYSIA)

HELAIAN MAKLUMAT PESAKIT

Anda dijemput untuk menyertai kajian ini. Sebelum menyertai kajian ini, sila baca dan fahami maklumat dalam dibentangkan di dalam Helaian Maklumat ini.

Tajuk kajian:
Penilaian tahap *liputan kesihatan sejagat* dalam pengurusan kanser payudara di Malaysia

Pengenalan:
Liputan kesihatan sejagat bermakna semua orang boleh mendapat semua perkhidmatan/rawatan, tanpa mengalami masalah kewangan semasa mendapatkan perkhidmatan/rawatan tersebut.

Tujuan kajian:
Kajian ini bertujuan untuk menilai rawatan kanser payudara di Malaysia dari segi *"liputan kesihatan sejagat"*.

Apa yang terlibat dalam kajian ini?
Peserta – pesakit kanser payudara yang menerima rawatan di hospital-hospital kerajaan.
Jika anda bersetuju untuk menyertai kajian ini – anda hanya perlu
   a) tandatangan "Borang Keizinan Pesakit", dan
   b) jawab beberapa soalan tentang rawatan yang anda jalani dan perbelanjaan yang anda tanggung semasa mendapat rawatan kanser payudara.

Risiko dan manfaat:
Risiko: Tiada risiko - kajian ini tidak boleh membahayakan diri anda atau menjejaskan rawatan anda.
Manfaat: Anda boleh membantu memberikan maklumat penting untuk membantu memperbaiki perkhidmatan/rawatan kanser payudara di Malaysia.

Adakah anda perlu mengambil bahagian?
Penyertaan dalam kajian ini adalah secara sukarela.
Anda boleh menarik diri dari kajian pada bila-bila masa, dan maklumat anda tidak akan digunakan.

Data & kerahsiaan:
Data kajian ini hanya boleh dibaca dan dikaji oleh penyelidik dan kumpulan yang bertanggungjawab di UKM (REC UKM).
Data ini akan dikaji secara keseluruhan, oleh itu maklumat anda secara perseorangan tidak akan didedahkan (kekal rahsia).
Setelah data ini dikaji ia akan dimasukkan ke dalam satu atau beberapa laporan.
Laporan-laporan tersebut akan dicetak atau diterbitkan.

Pembayaran dan pampasan:
Anda tidak perlu membayar untuk menyertai kajian ini.
Anda tidak akan dibayar untuk menyertai kajian ini.
Anda perlu membayar caj hospital seperti biasa jika anda mengambil bahagian dalam kajian ini.
Anda akan diberikan saguhati sebagai penghargaan atas penyertaan anda dalam kajian ini.

Siapa yang boleh saya tanya mengenai kajian ini?
Sebarang soalan boleh ditanya kepada Dr. Aidalina Mahmud di Jabatan Kesihatan Masyarakat, PPUKM (Tel: 03-91456986 / 012-3302158) atau REC PPUKM bagi mendapatkan penjelasan.

Penilaian tahap liputan kesihatan sejagat dalam pengurusan kanser payudara di Malaysia
Assessment of extent of universal health coverage in breast cancer management in Malaysia
Dr. Aidalina Mahmud 2015/2016 ©

Appendix B2

PATIENT INFORMATION SHEET (ENGLISH)

PATIENT INFORMATION SHEET

You are invited to participate in this study. Prior to participating in the study, please read and understand the information presented in this Information Sheet.

The title of the study:
Assessment of the extent of universal health coverage in the management of breast cancer in Malaysia.

Introduction:
Universal health coverage means everyone can get all services/treatment; without experiencing financial difficulties in getting the service/treatment.

The purpose of the study:
This study aims to evaluate the treatment of breast cancer in Malaysia in terms of *"universal health coverage"*.

What is involved in this study?
Participants - Breast cancer patients who receive treatment at government hospitals.
If you agree to participate in this study - you just have to
a) sign the "Patient Consent Form", and
b) answer a few questions about the treatment you undergo and the expenses you incur while receiving treatment for breast cancer.

Risks and benefits:
Risk: No risk - this study cannot endanger you or affect your treatment.
Benefit: You can help to provide important information to improve the services/treatment of breast cancer in Malaysia.

Do you need to participate?
Participation in this study is voluntary.
You can withdraw from the study at any time, and your information will not be used.

Data and confidentiality:
The survey data can only be read and studied by researchers and certain authorities (REC UKM).
Data will be analyzed as a whole, therefore your individual information will not be disclosed (they remain confidential).
Once the data is examined it will be included in one or several reports.
Such reports may be printed or published.

Payment and compensation:
You do not have to pay to participate in this study.
You will not be paid to participate in this study.
You have to pay hospital charges as usual if you participate in this study.
You will be given a token of appreciation for your participation in this study.

Who can I ask about the study?
Questions can be posed to Dr. Aidalina Mahmud at the Department of Community Health, PPUKM (Tel : 03-91456986 / 012-3392158) or REC PPUKM for clarification .

Appendix C1

DATA COLLECTION FORM

DATA COLLECTION FORM

ASSESSMENT OF THE EXTENT OF UNIVERSAL HEALTH COVERAGE IN BREAST CANCER MANAGEMENT IN MALAYSIA

COMPONENT TWO: SERVICE COVERAGE
(SERVICE UTILIZATION: REVIEW OF MEDICAL RECORDS)

	Value	Notes
ID		
Date of birth		
Diagnosis		
Date of diagnosis		MMG/HPE
Grade		
TNM		
Stage		
Nodes		node+ (four or more positive regional lymph nodes)
ER/PR/HER2		
FISH/DISH		
Date MMG		
Date surgery		MAC/BCS/Others
Date endocrine therapy		Tamox/ AI
Date radiotherapy		
Date targeted therapy		
Hospice/Palliative care		

Appendix C2

QUESTIONNAIRE

ASSESSMENT OF THE EXTENT OF UNIVERSAL HEALTH COVERAGE IN BREAST CANCER MANAGEMENT IN MALAYSIA

OUT-OF-POCKET EXPENDITURE FOR CANCER MANAGEMENT RELATIVE TO HOUSEHOLD NON-FOOD EXPENDITURE

Bahagian A. Sosio-demografi
Section A: Socio-demography

Arahan: Isikan tempat kosong dengan jawapan yang betul
Instructions: Fill in the blanks with the correct response.

No.	Item	Penerangan/Definition	Jawapan/Answer
1	Umur/ age	Umur semasa kajian dibuat berdasarkan tarikh lahir/ Age at time of study based on date of birth	
2	Kaum/ ethnicity		
3	Alamat rumah (ringkas) /home address (simplified)	Bandar & daerah tempat tinggal/ Town & district of residence	
4	Status perkahwinan/marital status	Status perkahwinan kini / Current marital status	Berkahwin/married Tidak berkahwin/single or separated or widowed
5	Tahap pengajian tertinggi /Highest education level		
6	Pekerjaan sebelum didiagnos kanser/ occupation prior to being diagnosed with cancer		
7	Pekerjaan selepas didiagnos kanser/ occupation after being diagnosed with cancer		
8	Komposisi isirumah/ Household composition	Bilangan, umur dan hubungan dengan pesakit/ Number, age and relationship with patient	
9	Adakah anda atau pasangan anda atau ibubapa anda penjawat awam?/ Are you, your spouse or your parents civil servants?	Untuk tahu samada layak menggunakan GL. To know if patient is eligible for GL use.	Ya/Yes Tidak/No
10	Adakah anda mempunyai insurans perubatan? /Do you have medical insurance?	Ya/Yes – Jika ya, ke soalan 4 dan 5 – If yes, to Q4 and 5 Tidak/No – Jika tidak, sila ke soalan 6 – If no, to Q6	Ya/Yes Tidak/No
11	Berapa premium insurans itu sebulan? / What is the premium per month?		RM
12	Adakah polisi insuran itu menampung kos rawatan kanser anda? Jika ya, berapa banyak? Does the health insurance policy cover the cost of your cancer treatment?If yes, how much		Ya/Yes Tidak/No *Perincian/details:

Bahagian B: Diagnosa dan rawatan
Section B: Diagnosis and treatment

No.	Item	Penerangan/Definition	Jawapan/Answer
1	Bila didiagnos kanser/ When diagnosed with cancer (date or approximate)		
2	Tahap kanser semasa didiagnosis/ Cancer stage at diagnosis		
3	Tahap kanser sekarang/ Cancer stage now		
4	Apakah rawatan kanser anda setakat ini? / What cancer treatment have you undergone so far?		
5	Di hospital anda mendapat rawatan setakat ini? / In which hospital have you received your cancer treatment so far?		
6	Setakat ini berapa kali anda pergi ke hospital/fasiliti kesihatan untuk hal berkaitan kanser? / So far, how many times did you go to the hospital/health facility for cancer related matters?	Investigation Clinic consultation Admission to ward	
7	Berapa bayaran untuk sekali rawatan pesakit luar? (purata) How much do you usually pay for an outpatient visit? (average)		RM _____
8	Pernahkah anda dimasukkan ke was setakat ini? Have you been admitted to the ward so far?	Ya/Yes – Jika ya, ke soalan 6 – If yes, to Q6 Tidak/No – Jika tidak, sila ke soalan 7 – If no, to Q7	Ya/Yes Tidak/No
9	Berapa kali anda dimasukkan ke wad dan berapa bayaran setiap kali kemasukan wad? How many times were you admitted into the ward and how much did you have to pay for each admission?		No.: _____ RM _____
10	Berapa anda perlu bayar untuk ubat berkaitan kanser, dalam sebulan? How much do you have to pay for medicines related to your cancer, in a month?	estimated household average monthly income and estimated household average monthly food expenditure	RM _____

Bahagian C: Anggaran pendapatan isirumah purata sebulan dan anggaran perbelajaan makanan isirumah sebulan
Section C: Estimated household average monthly income and estimated household average monthly food expenditure

No	Item	Penerangan/Definition	Jawapan/Answer
1.	Sumber pendapatan keluarga setiap bulan / *Source of family income, monthly*	Individu yang menyumbang pendapatan isirumah setiap bulan/ *Individuals who contribute to the household monthly income*	Diri sendiri/ *Self* = RM............ Suami/ *Husband* = RM............ Anak/ *Children* = RM............ Lain-lain/ *Others* = RM............
2.	Jumlah anggaran pendapatan bulanan dalam 12 bulan kebelakangan ini/ *Total average income per month in the last 12 months*	Jumlah anggaran pendapatan isirumah sebulan/ *Estimated amount of household income per month*	RM_____
3.	Adakah anda dibayar gaji atau mempunyai sumber pendapatan semasa menjalani rawatan kanser?/ *Do you still get your salary when undergoing cancer treatment?*	Ya/Yes – Jika ya, ke soalan 5 – *If yes, to Q5* Tidak/No – Jika tidak, sila ke soalan 4 – *If no, to Q4*	Ya/*Yes* Tidak/*No*
4.	Berapa banyak gaji dipotong / pengurangan pendapatan semasa anda menjalani rawatan kanser dalam 12 bulan yang lalu?/ *How much is your salary being cut/ reduction in your income while undergoing cancer treatment in the last 12 months?*		
5.	Anggaran perbelanjaan bulanan dapur (makan & minum) untuk isirumah sebulan. *Approximate monthly household expenditure for groceries (food & drinks)*	Raw food, Cooked food	RM_____

Bahagian D: Anggaran perbelajaan pengangkutan, makanan, tempat tinggal serta ubat tradisional dan komplimentari, sebulan
Section D: Estimated expenditure on travel, food, accommodation and traditional and complementary medicines, a month

No.	Item	Penerangan/Definition	Jawapan/Answer
1.	Apa jenis pengangkutan yang anda gunakan untuk ke hospital? / *What type of transportation do you use to go to hospital?*	Car Motorcycle Friend/ family Bus Taxi Combination private and public transport...	
2.	Berapa anggaran tambang pengangkutan awam untuk satu perjalanan pergi dan balik dari rumah ke hospital? / *What is the approximate fare for one trip to and from the hospital using public transportation?*		RM_____
3.	Berapa kali anda pergi dan/atau balik hospital menaiki kenderaan sendiri?/ *How many trips to and from the hospital which you used your own vehicle?* Hospital mana yang terlibat?/ *Which hospital was that?* Kenderaan jenis apa yang digunakan?/*What type of vehicle was used?*		
4.	Siapa temankan anda setiap kali anda ke hospital?/ *Who accompanies you to the hospital?*		RM_____
5.	Anggaran perbelanjaan makan & minum untuk orang yang menemani anda (jika ada) *Estimated expenses for food & drink for people who accompany you (if any)*	= approximate expenditure per meal x no. of meals per visit x no. of visits	
6.	Anggaran perbelanjaan penginapan untuk orang yang menemani anda (jika ada) *Estimated expenses for accommodation for people who accompany you (if any)*	= approximate expenditure per day of accommodation x no. of days per visit x no. of visits	
7.	Berapa banyak yang dibelanjakan sebulan (purata/anggaran) untuk ubat-ubatan komplementari dan supplementary (contoh: vitamin, rawatan tradisional dan sebagainya)/ *How much do you spend monthly (average/estimate) for*		

www.ingramcontent.com/pod-product-compliance
Lightning Source LLC
Chambersburg PA
CBHW020729180526
45163CB00001B/161